EMT-PARAMEDIC (P)

PRETEST® SELF-ASSESSMENT AND REVIEW

EMT-PARAMEDIC (P)

PRETEST® SELF-ASSESSMENT AND REVIEW

Richard E. J. Westfal, M.D., F.A.C.E.P.
Associate Director
Department of Emergency Medicine
Saint Vincent's Hospital
New York, New York
Associate Professor
Department of Emergency Medicine
New York Medical College
Valhalla, New York

John Filangeri, EMT-P
Paramedic Program Director
Hudson Valley Hospital Center
Peekskill, New York

Gregory Santa Maria, EMT-P
Paramedic Program Coordinator
Saint Vincent's Hospital
New York, New York

McGraw-Hill
Medical Publishing Division
PreTest® Series

New York   St. Louis   San Francisco   Auckland   Bogotá   Caracas   Lisbon   London   Madrid
Mexico City   Milan   Montreal   New Delhi   San Juan   Singapore   Sydney   Tokyo   Toronto

McGraw-Hill

*A Division of The **McGraw·Hill** Companies*

EMT-Paramedic (P): PreTest® Self-Assessment and Review

4 5 6 7 8 9 BKM BKM   0 9 8 7 6 5 4 3 2

ISBN 0-07-134156-0

This book was set in Times Roman by V&M Graphics.
The editors were John J. Dolan and Lester A. Sheinis.
The production supervisor was Minal Bopaiah.
Phoenix Book Technologies, Inc., was printer and binder.
The cover designer was Pinpoint Design.
The text designer was Robert Freese.

This book is printed on acid-free paper.

CONTENTS

PREFACE

Emergency Medical Technician–Paramedic: PreTest® Self-Assessment and Review has been created to prepare entry level and refresher Emergency Medical Technician-Paramedic (EMT-P) students for National Registry, regional, state, and city examinations. The book also is designed to assist EMT-P instructors, course coordinators, and medical directors to evaluate the progress of their students.

The United States Department of Transportation instituted a new curriculum for EMT-P training in 1994. The National Registry of Emergency Medical Technicians administers the EMT-P examinations, which are recognized by many states. All EMT-Ps are required to pass a written examination in order to be eligible to be certified or licensed to practice. Many states also administer their own written entry and rectification examinations every 3 to 4 years.

The new curriculum is divided into major modules, which include patient assessment, emergency medical services, scene assessment, trauma, pediatrics, and special situations. This review text is divided into sections, which correspond to each of the major modules. The total number of review questions is over 700. The questions are distributed among all of the study subjects, but emphasis is placed upon more questions for the critical emergencies than upon minor medical problems and administrative areas. The breakdown of the questions allows the student to evaluate his or her progress and to identify any areas of weakness, which may require additional study.

The majority of the questions are presented in the A-type multiple choice format. This format is the most frequently used in state and national certifying examinations. There is one correct answer and three distractors for each question. A brief rationale for the correct answer is given for each question. The questions are referenced to information included in the following textbooks: Brady's *Paramedic Emergency Care,* Caroline/Little Brown's *Emergency Care in the Streets,* Mosby/ACEPs *Paramedic Field Care,* and *Mosby's Paramedic Textbook.* Each answer has a chapter reference for the corresponding material in the textbook.

We all hope that this review text will assist each student in becoming a paramedic. We also hope that it will put some of the subjects in a clearer clinical light as well.

We would like to thank Lester Sheinis for his supervision of the editing of the text and our editor, John Dolan, for his steady support and guidance. Finally, we would like to thank our families and friends for their encouragement and patience.

Note

The bibliographic citations following each answer cite the publisher of the book first (Brady, Little Brown, Mosby, or Mosby/ACEP) and the section or chapter (e.g., Patient Assessment or Trauma) in that book in which relevant information can be found. For full book information on each citation, please see the Bibliography, on page 337.

EMT-PARAMEDIC (P)

PRETEST® SELF-ASSESSMENT AND REVIEW

SECTION I: PREPARATORY

The following topics are covered in Section I:

- Emergency Medical Services (EMS) Systems Roles and Responsibilities
- Well-Being of the Paramedic
- Medical Legal Issues
- Ethics
- Pharmacology
- Venous Access and Medication Administration

EMERGENCY MEDICAL SERVICES (EMS) SYSTEMS ROLES AND RESPONSIBILITIES

Directions: Each item below contains four suggested responses. Select the **one best** response to each item.

1. Match the following terms with the correct definitions:

   (A) EMS systems _____
   (B) licensure _____
   (C) professionalism _____
   (D) certification _____
   (E) profession _____
   (F) ethics _____
   (G) protocols _____
   (H) medical direction _____

   1. rules and standards that govern conduct
   2. conduct that characterizes a practitioner
   3. government agency verification of competency
   4. legal framework for Paramedics to act for doctors
   5. entity made up of personnel, equipment, and resources
   6. particular field or occupation
   7. standardized approach to common patient problems
   8. agency recognition of predetermined qualifications

2. All of the following are national groups that are important in the education and development of EMS EXCEPT

   (A) National Association of Emergency Medical Technicians (NAEMT)
   (B) National Association of EMS Physicians (NAEMSP)
   (C) Illinois State EMS Council
   (D) National Association of Search and Rescue (NASAR)

3. All of the following are the four nationally recognized levels of EMS training and education EXCEPT

   (A) First Responder
   (B) EMT-Basic
   (C) EMT-CC
   (D) EMT-Paramedic

4. In order to practice as a Paramedic, it is essential that you acquire which of the following?

(A) state certification and licensure
(B) national licensure
(C) Paramedic course completion
(D) county certification

5. All of the following are avenues for maintaining one's Paramedic competency through continuing medical education (CME) EXCEPT

(A) certification and recertification programs
(B) conferences and seminars
(C) independent study and journal review
(D) membership in national associations

6. All of the following functions are handled by the National Registry of Emergency Medical Technicians (NREMT) EXCEPT

(A) prepares and administers standardized tests for First Responder, EMT-Basic, EMT-Intermediate, and EMT-Paramedic
(B) assists in developing and evaluating EMT training programs
(C) provides national licensure
(D) works to establish a national minimum standard of competency for all of the levels of EMS training and education

7. Match all of the following examples of Paramedic professional behavior with the correct definition:

(A) integrity _____
(B) self-motivation _____
(C) communications _____
(D) time management _____
(E) self-confidence _____
(F) respect _____
(G) diplomacy _____
(H) patient advocacy _____

1. arriving to work on time and ready to go
2. presenting a case on telemetry
3. introducing yourself to each patient
4. persisting in having an emergently ill patient seen in the emergency department
5. calming your partner during argument with police
6. documenting your treatment on the call report
7. rapid ABCs assessment of the trauma victim
8. verbally taking control of treating an elderly patient with emotionally upset family members

8. You arrive at the scene where a 10-year-old male bicyclist has been hit by a car. Before you arrived on the scene, another EMS professional was dispatched to initiate emergency care. Which of the following BEST defines this person's role?

(A) family member
(B) First Responder
(C) EMT-Intermediate
(D) school nurse

9. All of the following are some of the responsibilities of the Paramedic EXCEPT

(A) scene size-up, communicating with dispatch
(B) allowing the EMT-Basic to assign patient care priorities
(C) initiating basic and advanced life support
(D) contact medical control

10. All of the following are correct statements concerning medical control EXCEPT

(A) involves only direct on-line communications with the Paramedic
(B) provides the legal framework for Paramedics to act on behalf of doctors
(C) includes providing reviewing calls with Paramedics and overseeing CME
(D) establishes and maintains prehospital protocols in conjunction with state and local laws

11. Which of the following is the main focus in providing quality improvement for an EMS system?

(A) ambulance maintenance
(B) billing procedures
(C) quality of supplies
(D) patient satisfaction

12. All of the following are correct concerning EMS research EXCEPT

(A) It is performed only by EMS physicians.
(B) It is an important part of any EMS system.
(C) Many Paramedic protocols and procedures have been instituted without clinical evidence of their safety or benefit to the patient.
(D) A research study consists of a hypothesis, literature review, study design, patient consent, and data collection, analysis, and statistical relevance.

EMERGENCY MEDICAL SERVICES (EMS) SYSTEMS ROLES AND RESPONSIBILITIES

A N S W E R S

1. **Answers.** (Brady, *Roles and Responsibilities of the Paramedic*. Caroline/Little Brown, *Roles and Responsibilities of the Paramedic.*)

   (A) 5
   (B) 3
   (C) 2
   (D) 8
   (E) 6
   (F) 1
   (G) 7
   (H) 4

2. **The answer is C.** (Brady, *Roles and Responsibilities of the Paramedic.*) Even though the organization in (C) may be very involved in state EMS education and development, it is not a national group. (A), (B), and (D) are all national groups.

3. **The answer is C.** (Mosby/ACEP, *Roles and Responsibilities.*) (A), (B), EMT-Intermediate, and (D) are the four nationally recognized levels of EMS training and education. (C) was formerly a level of EMS training and education; it has been replaced by EMT-Intermediate.

4. **The answer is A.** (Caroline/Little Brown, *Roles and Responsibilities of the Paramedic.*) Certification to practice as a Paramedic is granted at the state level. Many states require the Paramedic to pass the state EMT-Paramedic examination. However, many states accept the passing of the National Registry of Emergency Medical Technicians (NREMT) written and practical examination as an alternative. Most states also require recertification every 2 to 3 years. This may include a certain number of hours of CME as well.

5. The answer is D. (Mosby, *Roles and Responsibilities.*) (A), (B), (C), lectures and work-shops, quality-improvement case reviews, skill laboratories, videotape reviews, and approved computer Internet courses are some of the well-accepted methods of acquiring CME for maintaining Paramedic competency. (D) is not considered CME, even though participation in national associations is considered to be professionally important.

6. The answer is C. (Brady, *Roles and Responsibilities of the Paramedic.*) (A), (B), (D), and serves as a widely accepted manner of providing reciprocity for EMS professionals seeking to move and practice in a new state. (C) is not a function of the NREMT because licensure and certification are granted on the state level. However, many states are accepting NREMT certification as an alternative.

7. Answers. (Mosby, *Roles and Responsiblities.*)

(A) 6
(B) 1
(C) 2
(D) 7
(E) 8
(F) 3
(G) 5
(H) 4

8. The answer is B. (Mosby, *Roles and Responsibilities.*) (A), (C), and (D) are incorrect. First Responder best defines the role, even though any of the other individuals, with proper training, could act in this capacity.

9. The answer is B. (Brady, *Roles and Responsibilities of the Paramedic.*) (A), (C), (D), conducting patient assessments, communicating with other team members, assessing the results of treatment, directing and coordinating transport, and maintaining rapport with the patient, support agencies, and the hospital are all some of the responsibilities of the Paramedic. (B) is incorrect because the EMT-Paramedic, having advanced training, is responsible to assign patient care priorities, not the EMT-Basic. However, it is essential to properly use the skills and capabilities of all emergency personnel on the scene.

10. The answer is A. (Caroline/Little Brown, *Roles and Responsibilities of the Paramedic.*) (B), (C), and (D) are correct statements. Statement (A) is incorrect because, while medical control does involve direct on-line medical control communications, it also involves many off-line responsibilities, including quality assurance and continuing quality improvement, providing call-review sessions, arranging and providing CME, participating with local pre-hospital community committees, and in-servicing telemetry physicians.

11. **The answer is D.** (Brady, *Emergency Medical Services Systems.*) (A), (B), and (C) are incorrect, because, even though these may be some of the areas to follow in assessing quality improvement, patient satisfaction is truly the top priority.

12. **The answer is A.** (Brady, *Emergency Medical Services Systems.*) (B), (C), and (D) are correct statements. Statement (A) is incorrect, because, even though EMS physicians may be involved in EMS research, all prehospital providers are encouraged to participate in EMS research, with or without EMS physician participation.

WELL-BEING OF THE PARAMEDIC

Directions: Each item below contains four suggested responses. Select the **one best** response to each item.

13. Which of the following is the BEST definition of wellness?

 (A) simply feeling good
 (B) being free of any known medical illnesses
 (C) the concept that encourages people to take responsibility for their health
 (D) the practice of treating patients and making them well

14. All of the following are components of wellness EXCEPT

 (A) physical well-being
 (B) financial well-being
 (C) mental and emotional well-being
 (D) spiritual well-being

15. All of the following are examples of wellness programs EXCEPT

 (A) smoking cessation
 (B) weight reduction
 (C) stress management
 (D) home repair course

16. All of the following are parts of the three stages of stress EXCEPT

 (A) alarm
 (B) resistance
 (C) exhaustion
 (D) overreaction

17. All of the following are factors that may trigger a stress response EXCEPT

 (A) complimentary letter
 (B) personal injury
 (C) loss of a loved one
 (D) job stress

18. In dealing with a stressful situation, a Paramedic may experience detrimental anxiety levels. All of the following are symptoms of anxiety EXCEPT

(A) palpitations
(B) anorexia, nausea, vomiting, and abdominal cramps
(C) high, persistent fever
(D) headache

19. You are dispatched to a 45-year-old male who is emotionally disturbed and is in possible possession of a weapon. You are the first to arrive at the scene and can clearly see through the front window of the house that the patient is screaming and has a large knife in his hand. All of the following are parts of the approach to dealing with this patient EXCEPT

(A) Immediately introduce yourself, enter the house, and begin to softly calm the patient down.
(B) Avoid verbal confrontation with the patient and try to listen to him.
(C) Avoid allowing the patient to block the exit.
(D) Before attempting to restrain a patient, make sure that adequate help is available.

20. All of the following are defense mechanisms that individuals commonly use to deal with stress EXCEPT

(A) denial
(B) rationalization
(C) isolation
(D) crying

21. You have been working in your ambulance department for the past 7 years and have noticed that one of your co-workers has been steadily demonstrating signs and symptoms of "burnout." He has been less interested in his work, arriving late to work frequently, complaining about the system regularly, drinking more at night, and having increasing difficulty dealing with his friends and family. Which of the following is the correct definition for this condition?

(A) acute stress reaction
(B) cumulative stress
(C) critical incident stress
(D) delayed stress

22. You are sent to a bomb explosion at a nearby school. As you arrive, you are told that the fire and police departments have confirmed that the scene is currently safe. You are also told that there are over 50 serious injuries and several deaths. As you and your fellow EMS providers, police, and fire fighters begin to enter the scene, an incident commander is already beginning to plan to assist all responders with the critical incident stress associated with this disaster. All of the following are possible parts of the on-scene critical incident stress management EXCEPT

(A) briefing rescuers about what to expect before deployment to the scene
(B) providing 15- to 20-minute breaks every 2 hours, away from the scene
(C) calling all of the emergency responders together 1 hour into the event for a 30-minute talk
(D) ensuring that maximum exposure on the scene does not exceed 12 hours

23. All of the following are some of the techniques used by critical incident stress management teams to help the emergency responders deal with the stress EXCEPT

(A) demobilization
(B) debriefing
(C) referral
(D) denial

24. According to a study by Dr. Elisabeth Kübler-Ross, *On Death and Dying*, all of the following are stages of the grieving process EXCEPT

(A) denial
(B) anger
(C) exhilaration
(D) depression

25. All of the following affect the individual Paramedic's attitude toward death and dying EXCEPT

(A) religious and cultural understanding
(B) prejudices
(C) your grandmother's death, before you were born
(D) prior experiences

WELL-BEING OF THE PARAMEDIC

ANSWERS

13. **The answer is C.** (Mosby/ACEP, *Stress and Stress Management.*) Wellness is based on the premise that people have control over their health behaviors. (A), (B), and (D) are incorrect.

14. **The answer is B.** (Mosby/ACEP, *Stress and Stress Management.*) (A), (C), and (D) are components of wellness. (B) is not.

15. **The answer is D.** (Mosby/ACEP, *Stress and Stress Management.*) (A), (B), (C), cholesterol and blood pressure screening, nutrition, physical fitness, and safety education are examples of wellness programs. (D) is not.

16. **The answer is D.** (Brady, *Stress Management in Emergency Services.*) (A), (B), and (C) are the classic three stages of stress. (D) is not a stage of stress.

17. **The answer is A.** (Caroline/Little Brown, *Stress Management.*) (B), (C), (D), and any major life events are some examples of stress triggers. (A) is not a stress trigger because a complimentary letter usually brings about a positive and comforting feeling.

18. **The answer is C.** (Brady, *Stress Management in Emergency Services.*) (A), (B), (D), rapid or difficult breathing, dry mouth, chest tightness, sweating, flushing, urinary frequency, and muscle or joint aches are some of the symptoms of anxiety. (C) is not a symptom of anxiety because, even though anxiety may trigger fluctuations in body temperature, it should not produce a persistently high fever. A physical examination looking for a possible infectious cause would be in order.

19. The answer is A. (Mosby/ACEP, *Issues of Personal Violence.*) (B), (C), and (D) are all correct. (A) is incorrect because, at a violent scene, scene safety must first be established by the police. It would be a serious mistake to enter the home of this emotionally disturbed patient before the police have established scene safety.

20. The answer is D. (Mosby, *Stress Management.*) (A), (B), (C), compensation, reaction formation, substitution, sublimation, regression, repression, and projection are all some of the defense mechanisms used to deal with stress. (D) is incorrect because crying may be an outward expression of stress but is not considered a defense mechanism.

21. The answer is B. (Mosby/ACEP, *Stress and Stress Management.*) Cumulative stress reactions are the result of multiple stresses occurring over time. Physical and emotional exhaustion and negative attitudes characterize it. (A), (C), and (D) are incorrect. An acute stress reaction is immediate and incident specific. Critical incident stress is the reaction that many emergency-responding individuals have to a disaster or multicasualty incident. Delayed stress reactions are also the result of a specific incident, but the Paramedic may not experience symptoms until days, months, or years later.

22. The answer is C. (Mosby/ACEP, *Stress and Stress Management.*) (A), (B), (D), allowing completion of tasks before changing assignments, integrating veterans to teach newcomers how to perform the task, providing meals and snacks, maintaining normal working groups, and providing decaffeinated beverages are some of the skills used to deal with critical incident stress. (C) is not used because it would be unwise and impossible to remove all emergency responders together from the event in order to talk to them. During the event, such a response may result in more casualties and would add to the critical incident stress for the responders.

23. The answer is D. (Mosby/ACEP, *Stress and Stress Management.*) (A), (B), (C), and defusing are some of the techniques used. (D) is incorrect because, while denial is one of the defense mechanisms an individual may use to deal with stress, it is not a technique used by critical incident stress management teams. Rather, the correct approach is to try to assist the EMS responder with expressing his or her feelings concerning the entire experience.

24. The answer is C. (Caroline/Little Brown, *Stress Management.* Brady, *Stress Management in Emergency Services.*) (A), (B), (D), bargaining, and acceptance are the five stages of the grieving process. (C) is incorrect.

25. The answer is C. (Mosby/ACEP, *Death and Dying.*) (A), (B), and (D) play an integral part in affecting each Paramedic's attitude toward death and dying. (C) does not because your grandmother's death, occurring before you were born, would have little affect upon your own personal feelings toward death and dying.

MEDICAL LEGAL ISSUES

Directions: Each item below contains four suggested responses. Select the **one best** response to each item.

26. Your Paramedic unit is assigned to a call for an asthmatic. On your arrival, you find a 27-year-old known asthmatic who is complaining of severe difficulty breathing. You assess and begin treatment, including advanced life support care. While you are treating this patient, your partner states that the police department is calling for an ambulance for a confirmed shooting only three blocks away. You and your partner pack up your equipment and tell the patient that he should be OK, and you respond to the shooting. Later you find out that the patient called for another ambulance an hour later and was intubated by the Paramedics. In addition to abandonment, you may also be charged with which of the following?

(A) assault
(B) negligence
(C) slander
(D) libel

27. You are assigned to an unconscious patient who is a known diabetic. After your assessment, you administer oxygen and 50 percent dextrose intravenously (IV). The patient awakens and is transported to the hospital without incident. You initially treated this patient under which type of consent?

(A) informed
(B) implied
(C) involuntary
(D) assumed

28. Match the following statements with their definitions

    (A) abandonment _____
    (B) battery _____
    (C) assault _____
    (D) libel _____
    (E) slander _____
    (F) false imprisonment _____

1. damaging a patient's character by using false or malicious spoken terms
2. damaging a patient's character by using false or malicious written terms
3. committing an act that places the patient in fear of bodily harm
4. termination of a patient's care prior to ensuring a continuation of proper care
5. touching a patient against his or her consent
6. intentionally and unjustifiably detaining a patient against his or her will

29. The Paramedic may be required to report all of the following types of cases to the proper authorities EXCEPT

    (A) child abuse
    (B) gunshot wounds
    (C) myocardial infarction in a 28-year-old female
    (D) rape

30. You are treating a 70-year-old patient whose family contacted EMS because the patient was experiencing chest pain. On your arrival, the patient is in obvious distress. The patient states that he has been in the hospital too much lately and will not go back. Although you attempt numerous times to convince the patient to go to the hospital, he adamantly refuses. All of the following should be documented on your call report EXCEPT

    (A) patient's name, address, and date of birth
    (B) vital signs and Paramedic interventions
    (C) attempts to convince the patient to change his mind
    (D) Nothing should be written on the report, since the patient is refusing transport.

MEDICAL LEGAL ISSUES

ANSWERS

26. The answer is B. (Mosby, *Medical-Legal Considerations.*) The charge of negligence is proven when four criteria are met. Based on the scenario, you and your partner have met the following criteria to be charged with negligence: (1) Based on the fact that you were being compensated for your treatment (paid Paramedic), you had a duty to act, since you were assigned to the call. (2) Your conduct was not reasonable or expected behavior. (3) Your leaving the patient without further assessment or transport caused additional damage to the patient's condition. (4) Your abandonment of the patient was the proximate cause of his deterioration. Although it may be argued that the Paramedic crew did not injure the patient, in this case, inappropriate treatment was the cause of this patient's deterioration. (A), (C), and (D), are incorrect.

27. The answer is B. (Brady, *Medical Legal Considerations of Emergency Care.*) (B) is correct, since the patient was unconscious. The definition of implied consent states that if the patient were conscious and able to agree to care, they would have allowed you to treat them. (A) Informed consent applies to the conscious patient who makes a decision to be treated after an explanation of the diagnosis and the possible treatments. (C) Involuntary consent usually involves a court order to initiate care of the patient. (D) is incorrect.

28. Answers. (Brady, *Medical Legal Considerations of Emergency Care.*)
- (A) 4
- (B) 5
- (C) 3
- (D) 2
- (E) 1
- (F) 6

29. The answer is C. (Mosby, *Medical-Legal Considerations.*) Paramedics may be required by law to report all types of injuries that may be the result of criminal activity. All of the answers are correct with the exception of (C). Although it may seem odd that a 28-year-old female would be having a myocardial infarction, it is indeed not criminal. Paramedics may also be required to report certain instances of illness and/or communicable diseases.

30. The answer is D. (Mosby, *Medical-Legal Considerations.*) Many lawsuits arise out of patients' refusal of care. Paramedics need to be especially careful about the documentation of these patients. All patient interactions should be thoroughly documented. (A), (B), and (C) are all pertinent pieces of information that must be documented. In addition, the Paramedic should have the refusal signed by the patient and witnessed by family members or a member of law enforcement.

ETHICS

Directions: Each item below contains four suggested responses. Select the **one best** response to each item.

31. Which of the following is the BEST definition of ethics?

(A) simple compliance to peer pressure
(B) the study of standards, conduct, and moral judgment that governs the conduct of members of a particular group
(C) following orders, right or wrong
(D) religious teachings that affect any given person

32. Which of the following is the BEST premise to underlie the Paramedic's ethical decisions in the prehospital environment?

(A) Place the welfare of the patient ahead of all other considerations.
(B) Intervene only when you feel that it is correct to do so.
(C) Follow the family's wishes regardless of your protocols or state statutes.
(D) Follow your partner's decisions on any difficult situation.

33. You are dispatched to the scene of a 97-year-old male who has just lost consciousness. As you walk into the home, a crying family member informs you that the patient has been dying for the past 6 months of widespread cancer. As you approach the patient, you note that he is breathing 8 times per minute, his pulse is 30 beats per minute, and his blood pressure is 50 palpable. There are no signs of trauma and no indications of foul play. For a Paramedic, which of the following is the most reasonable approach to this patient?

(A) Immediately intubate, force IV fluids, and consider an external pacemaker.

(B) Knowing your state law and your EMS system rules and regulations concerning advanced directives, inquire of the patient's family members whether there are any such advanced directives in effect, and proceed according to a combination of the laws, rules, and directives.

(C) Do not treat this patient until you have personally spoken to his physician and your own medical control.

(D) Follow your heart and try to avoid any treatment of this patient at any cost.

ETHICS

ANSWERS

31. The answer is B. (Brady, *Roles and Responsibilities of the Paramedic*. Mosby, *Roles and Responsibilities*.) (A), (C), and (D) are incorrect because, even though each may play a part in the practice of the Paramedic, none is a part of the definition of ethics.

32. The answer is A. (Caroline/Little Brown, *Medicolegal and Ethical Issues*.) (B), (C), and (D) are incorrect.

33. This answer is B. (Mosby/ACEP, *Death and Dying*.) Even in trying to keep the patient's best interests in mind, you must be familiar with your state law and your EMS system rules and regulations concerning advanced directives. If the present situation is a little confusing, you may choose to contact medical control in order to have additional input on how to proceed. In the meantime, even if you have been directed to honor any advanced directives, you should still provide comfort care for the patient and emotional support for the family member.

PHARMACOLOGY

Directions: Each item below contains four suggested responses. Select the **one best** response to each item.

34. The description of a drug using its chemical name and molecular structure is the

(A) trade name
(B) official name
(C) chemical name
(D) brand name

35. Demerol Hydrochloride is an example of a

(A) chemical name
(B) generic name
(C) trade name
(D) official name

36. Which of the following drugs is derived from a plant?

(A) lidocaine hydrochloride
(B) magnesium sulfate
(C) penicillin
(D) digitalis

37. Bretylium tosylate, lidocaine, and procainamide are all examples of medications derived from

(A) plants
(B) minerals
(C) animals
(D) synthetics

the following are accepted publi-
ca...s on drug information EXCEPT

(A) medical dictionaries
(B) American Medical Association
(AMA) drug evaluation
(C) medication package inserts
(D) *Physicians' Desk Reference*

39. A controlled substance that is classified
as schedule I is defined as a drug with

(A) high abuse potential and accepted
medical uses
(B) moderate abuse potential and
accepted medical uses
(C) low abuse potential and accepted
medical uses
(D) high abuse potential and no medical
uses

40. You respond to an unconscious patient
in a park. On your arrival you find a
23-year-old male who is unresponsive.
His companion is on the scene and
states that the patient had injected heroin
as well as "taken some Valium" prior to
losing consciousness. The history provided by his companion leads you to
conclude that the patient has overdosed
on medications classified as

(A) schedule II and schedule IV
(B) schedule III and schedule I
(C) schedule IV and schedule II
(D) schedule I and schedule IV

41. Pharmacokinetics can BEST be
described as

(A) a drug's mechanism of action upon
the body
(B) a drug's affect on the receptor sites
(C) the entry of medications into the
body and their elimination
(D) the use of medications in trauma
patients

42. Pharmacodynamics can BEST be
described as

(A) biotransformation to convert a drug
into an active form
(B) the process in which the desired
biochemical response is achieved
(C) the elimination of a drug through
metabolism
(D) the crossing of a medication
through the blood-brain barrier

43. All of the following are pharmacokinetic
factors EXCEPT

(A) absorption
(B) distribution
(C) elimination
(D) therapeutic index

44. Your patient is taking a beta agonist, a
medication that will

(A) stimulate an increase in beta activ-
ity, creating a desired drug effect
(B) inhibit beta activity by blocking
receptor sites
(C) biotransform his beta medication
(D) energize the target tissue

45. Your patient is suspected of taking an
overdose of an opioid derivative. In
order to reverse this overdose, you
should administer a

(A) narcotic agonist
(B) narcotic antagonist
(C) benzodiazepine agonist
(D) benzodiazepine antagonist

46. Your 35-year-old female patient has overdosed on diazepam and is unconscious. Flumazenil is administered, and the patient begins to stir and become more oriented to her surroundings. Flumazenil is an example of a

(A) narcotic agonist
(B) narcotic antagonist
(C) benzodiazepine agonist
(D) benzodiazepine antagonist

47. Liquid penicillin is an example of which drug form?

(A) emulsion
(B) fluid extract
(C) elixir
(D) suspension

48. Your patient has self-administered sublingual nitroglycerin for his chest pain. Nitroglycerin is an example of which type of solid drug?

(A) pill
(B) powder
(C) tablet
(D) capsule

49. Elixirs, emulsions, suspensions, and solutions are all examples of which form of drug?

(A) liquid
(B) solid
(C) parenteral
(D) spirits

50. The term potentiation is used to describe which of the following circumstances?

(A) the enhancement of the effect of one drug by another drug
(B) an effect in which the absence of a drug causes physical or emotional disturbances
(C) the effect gained by taking multiple doses of a single drug
(D) two drugs, administered together, whose total effect equals the sum of the effects of each individual agent

51. A side effect of a drug that produces an outcome harmful to the patient is called a

(A) contraindication
(B) untoward effect (reaction)
(C) depressant
(D) therapeutic action

52. Most drugs have known and expected side effects. However, in certain patients, a drug may have a side effect that is neither known nor expected. This circumstance is defined as

(A) idiosyncracy
(B) synergism
(C) potentiation
(D) tolerance

53. The administration of a drug in several doses, causing an increased effect due to a buildup of the drug in the blood, is called

(A) antagonism
(B) cumulative action
(C) idiosyncratic reaction
(D) therapeutic action

54. Your patient has been taking a medication for several years. The patient tells you that, over the years, his physician has kept increasing the dosage when the drug has stopped working as well at the old dosage. This situation is known as

(A) habituation
(B) synergism
(C) antagonism
(D) tolerance

55. The process by which a drug is converted into an active form in the blood or body tissue is called

(A) absorption
(B) distribution
(C) biotransformation
(D) elimination

56. All of the following are responsible for the excretion of drug metabolites EXCEPT

(A) kidneys
(B) liver
(C) intestines
(D) lungs

57. You administer 100 mg of a medication with a half-life of 2 hours. How many hours will it take for the medication to be excreted to less than 1 mg?

(A) 10 hours
(B) 12 hours
(C) 14 hours
(D) 16 hours

58. A medication that would produce the same effect as that of the sympathetic nervous system is known as

(A) sympathomimetic
(B) sympatholytic
(C) parasympathomimetic
(D) parasympatholytic

59. All of the following drugs are sympathomimetics EXCEPT

(A) lidocaine
(B) epinephrine
(C) dopamine
(D) norepinephrine (Levophed)

60. All of the following are classified as benzodiazepines EXCEPT

(A) flumazenil
(B) lorazepam
(C) diazepam
(D) midazolam

61. Of the following medications, which is NOT classified as an antidysrhythmic agent?

(A) lidocaine
(B) procainamide
(C) magnesium sulfate
(D) bretylium tosylate

62. All of the following are parenteral routes of drug administration EXCEPT

(A) IV
(B) endotracheal
(C) intramuscular
(D) rectal

63. Arrange, in order from fastest to slowest, the rates of drug absorption for different routes of drug administration:

(A) intramuscular
(B) endotracheal
(C) IV
(D) sublingual
(E) oral
(F) subcutaneous

1. 1, 4, 2, 3, 6, 5
2. 2, 4, 3, 1, 6, 5
3. 3, 2, 1, 6, 4, 5
4. 4, 6, 3, 1, 2, 5

PHARMACOLOGY

A N S W E R S

34. The answer is C. (Mosby, *Emergency Pharmacology.*) (C) The chemical name of a drug is a precise description of its chemical composition and molecular structure. Although (A), (B), and (D) are also used in the description of drugs, trade names are the copyrighted names given by the drug manufacturer, official names are the listings in the United States Pharmacopoeia or National Formulary, and brand name, the proprietary name, is another term for trade name.

35. The answer is C. (Mosby, *Emergency Pharmacology.*) (C) Demerol Hydrochloride is the trade name for meperidine hydrochloride. It is a potent narcotic analgesic. The trade name is the copyrighted name given by the drug manufacturer. (A), (B), and (D) are incorrect.

36. The answer is D. (Mosby, *Emergency Pharmacology.*) (D) Digitalis is a derivative of the foxglove plant. There are five classifications of drug derivatives: plants (e.g., atropine sulfate, digitalis, and morphine sulfate), chemical substances (e.g., lidocaine), minerals (e.g., sodium bicarbonate and calcium chloride), microorganisms (e.g., penicillin), and animals and humans (e.g., insulin and epinephrine).

37. The answer is D. (Brady, *Emergency Pharmacology.*) (D) Bretylium tosylate, lidocaine, and procainamide are all synthetic medications. These medications have been developed in drug laboratories and are not natural derivatives. (A), (B), and (C) are incorrect.

38. The answer is A. (Mosby, *Emergency Pharmacology.*) (A) Medical dictionaries do not contain comprehensive drug information. (B) The AMA drug evaluation, (C) medication package inserts, and (D) the Physicians' Desk Reference are considered good resources of drug information for the Paramedic. The Hospital Formulary is also a good reference for drug information.

39. The answer is D. (Mosby, *Emergency Pharmacology.*) Schedule I drugs are classified as illegal drugs of abuse (e.g., heroin, mescaline, and LSD); they have high abuse potential and no accepted medical uses. Schedule II drugs (e.g., opiates and amphetamines) have high abuse potential but positive medical benefits. Schedule III drugs, which contain limited quantities of schedule II drugs, have a lower abuse potential than do schedule I and II medications. Schedule IV drugs (e.g., phenobarbital and diazepam) have a lower abuse potential than do schedule I, II, and III drugs. Schedule V drugs contain limited quantities of certain opioids and are generally used in cough or diarrhea control.

40. The answer is D. (Mosby, *Emergency Pharmacology.*) Heroin is a schedule I drug with no accepted medical uses, while diazepam (Valium) is a schedule IV medication with accepted medical uses. Schedule I medications are not available by prescription. Schedule IV medications are available by a physician prescription only. These prescriptions have strict guidelines that control the amount of refills as well as the length that the prescription may be refilled. All schedule II, III, and IV medications must carry warning labels that alert the user to their abuse potential.

41. The answer is C. (Brady, *Emergency Pharmacology.*) (C) Pharmacokinetics is the study of how a drug enters the body and reaches its site of action. It includes absorption, distribution, biotransformation, and subsequent elimination through metabolism. (A), (B), and (D) are incorrect.

42. The answer is B. (Brady, *Emergency Pharmacology.*) (B) Pharmacodynamics is the process in which a drug binds to a receptor on the cell membrane and initiates a biochemical reaction, creating the desired response. (A), biotransformation, is the process by which a drug is made active or inactive. (C), the elimination of a drug, is part of the metabolic process of the body (pharmacokinetics). (D), the crossing of the blood-brain barrier, is part of the distribution process (pharmacokinetics).

43. The answer is D. (Brady, *Emergency Pharmacology.*) (D) The therapeutic index is the difference between the toxic and the effective dose of a medication. Therapeutic index is a factor of pharmacodynamics (the induction of a biochemical response). (A), (B), and (C) are all pharmacokinetic factors.

44. The answer is A. (Brady, *Emergency Pharmacology.*) (A) A beta agonist attaches to the cell's receptor site (a protein on the cell that allows a drug to bind to it) and creates the desired effect of the drug. The process described in (B), the inhibition of the binding of one drug by another, is called antagonism. (C) and (D) are also incorrect.

45. The answer is B. (Mosby, *Emergency Pharmacology.*) (B) To reverse the effects of an opioid derivative, the Paramedic should administer an opioid antagonist, in this case, naloxone. Naloxone competes for the opiate receptor sites and eliminates the effects of the opiate. (A) A narcotic agonist would stimulate receptors, thereby increasing the opioid effect.

(C) A benzodiazepine agonist would potentiate the effects of the opioid by adding its sedative-hypnotic effect to the opioid overdose. (D) A benzodiazepine antagonist would have no effect on an opioid.

46. The answer is D. (Mosby, *Emergency Drug Index.*) (D) Flumazenil is a benzodiazepine receptor antagonist. A receptor antagonist blocks the receptor site of certain drugs, rendering their mechanism of action ineffective. (A) A narcotic agonist, such as morphine sulfate, would attach to the receptor and create a narcotic effect. (B) A narcotic antagonist, such as naloxone (Narcan), is incorrect because flumazenil, although an agonist itself, will not block the receptor sites for narcotics. (C) A benzodiazepine receptor agonist would be an actual benzodiazepine, such as diazepam or lorazepam; this patient has overdosed on this type of agonist.

47. The answer is D. (Caroline/Little Brown, *Overview of Pharmacology.*) (D) A suspension is a drug (usually a powder) that is added to a liquid to facilitate oral administration. Penicillin, although available in solid form, is commonly administered to children in a liquid form. Suspensions have a tendency to separate and therefore require shaking before administration. (A) Emulsions are usually oil-and-water mixtures that are used, for example, as lubricants. (B) A fluid extract is a drug that is readily soluble in a particular fluid. (C) An elixir is a syrup with the addition of alcohol.

48. The answer is C. (Caroline/Little Brown, *Overview of Pharmacology.*) (C) Nitroglycerin comes in several forms, but only (C) is correct in this instance. (A), (B), and (D) are incorrect. (A) Pills are drugs shaped in an easy-to-swallow form. (B) Powders are drugs that have been crushed and combined with other powders to form a mixture. (D) Capsules are gelatin containers that hold a dose of medication, usually in powder form.

49. The answer is A. (Brady, *Emergency Pharmacology.*) (A) Liquid drugs include solutions, tinctures, suspensions, spirits, emulsions, elixirs, and syrups. (B) Solid drugs include pills, powders, capsules, tablets, and suppositories. (C) Parenteral drugs are liquid drugs that are administered through intramuscular, subcutaneous, or intravenous routes. (D) Spirits are considered a liquid drug.

50. The answer is A. (Mosby, *Emergency Pharmacology.*) (A) Potentiation is the enhancement of a drug's effect when concurrently administered with another drug (e.g., alcohol and barbiturates). (B), (C), and (D) are incorrect; they describe drug dependency, cumulative action, and synergism, respectively.

51. The answer is B. (Mosby, *Emergency Pharmacology.*) (B) An untoward effect (reaction) is a side effect that produces a harmful outcome for the patient. Certain harmful side effects may be listed as contraindications. (A) A contraindication is a condition that could result in a dangerous outcome with the administration of the medication. (C) Depressants decrease body functions and activities. (D) Therapeutic action is the desired effect of a given drug.

52. The answer is A. (Brady, *Emergency Pharmacology.*) (A) An idiosyncratic reaction is an individual reaction to a drug that is not a usually expected reaction. (B), (C), and (D) are incorrect.

53. The answer is B. (Brady, *Emergency Pharmacology.*) (B) Cumulative action occurs when a drug is administered in several doses; the buildup of the drug in the bloodstream causes an increased therapeutic effect. (A), (C), and (D) are incorrect.

54. The answer is D. (Mosby, *Emergency Pharmacology.*) (D) Tolerance is the effect that occurs when a patient taking a long-term medication needs to have its dosage increased to maintain the therapeutic effect. Tolerance is caused by a decreased physiological response to a drug administered long term. (A) Habituation is physical or psychological dependence on a drug. (B) Synergism is the combined action of two drugs that exceeds the sum of the actions of each individual drug. (C) Antagonism is opposition between the effects of two agents in which one overtakes the receptor sites of the other, creating a drug blockade.

55. The answer is C. (Brady, *Emergency Pharmacology.*) (C) Biotransformation occurs when a drug is administered and it is converted into an active or inactive form. This usually occurs in the blood or body tissues. (A) Absorption refers to the absorption of drugs into the capillary beds. (B) Distribution is the delivery of a drug to its proper receptor site via the bloodstream. (D) Elimination is the breakdown of a drug and its subsequent elimination from the body, usually in the form of metabolites.

56. The answer is B. (Mosby, *Emergency Pharmacology.*) (B) The liver, although responsible for the metabolism of many medications, is not directly responsible for their excretion. The (A) kidneys, (C) intestines, and (D) lungs accomplish drug metabolite excretion. Sweat and salivary glands are also responsible for drug metabolite excretion, but at a lesser level of importance.

57. The answer is C. (Mosby, *Emergency Pharmacology.*) (C) 14 hours is correct. To figure out the excretion rate of this medication, you would divide the dosage in half at every 2-hour interval. In this case, it would take 14 hours for the medication to drop below 1 mg. (A), (B), and (D) are incorrect.

58. The answer is A. (Brady, *Emergency Pharmacology.*) (A) Sympathomimetics are drugs or other substances that produce effects like those of the sympathetic nervous system. (B) Sympatholytics are drugs or other substances that block the sympathetic nervous system. (C) Parasympathomimetics cause effects like those of the parasympathetic nervous system. (D) Parasympatholytics are drugs or other substances that block the parasympathetic nervous system (e.g., atropine).

59. The answer is A. (Brady, *Emergency Pharmacology.*) (A) Lidocaine is classified as an antidysrhythmic medication. (B) Epinephrine, (C) dopamine, and (D) norepinephrine (Levophed) are all classified as sympathomimetics or sympathetic agonists.

60. The answer is A. (Mosby, *Emergency Drug Index.*) (A) Flumazenil is a benzodiazepine antagonist and is commonly administered to counteract an overdose of benzodiazepines. (B) Lorazepam (Ativan), (C) diazepam (Valium), and (D) midazolam (Versed) are all benzodiazepines. These medications are also known as sedative-hypnotics.

61. The answer is C. (Brady, *Emergency Pharmacology.*) (C) Magnesium sulfate, although used in the treatment of dysrhythmias, is classified as an electrolyte and/or central nervous system depressant. It is an essential element in many of the biochemical reactions that occur in the body. (A) Lidocaine, (B) procainamide, and (D) bretylium tosylate are all classified as antidysrhythmics.

62. The answer is D. (Mosby, *Emergency Pharmacology.*) (D) The rectal route of drug administration is called an enteral route. Enteral routes include oral, gastric, small intestinal, and rectal. Enteral routes are the safest routes of drug administration; they are also the most unreliable. (A) Intravenous, (B) endotracheal, and (C) intramuscular are all parenteral routes.

63. The answer is C. (Caroline/Little Brown, *Overview of Pharmacology.*) (C) 3, 2, 1, 6, 4, 5 is the correct order of absorption. The actual order, including all routes of administration, is intracardiac, intravenous, endotracheal, inhalation, sublingual, intramuscular, subcutaneous, rectal, oral, and topical.

VENOUS ACCESS AND MEDICATION ADMINISTRATION

Directions: Each item below contains four suggested responses. Select the **one best** response to each item.

64. All of the following drugs may be administered endotracheally EXCEPT

(A) lidocaine
(B) furosemide
(C) epinephrine
(D) atropine

65. You are ordered to administer 5 mL of a 4 percent medication. How many milligrams should you administer to the patient?

(A) 20 mg
(B) 50 mg
(C) 100 mg
(D) 200 mg

66. Your medical control physician orders you to administer 80 mg of furosemide. Furosemide is supplied in vials that contain 40 mg in 4 mL. How many milliliters should you administer?

(A) 2 mL
(B) 4 mL
(C) 6 mL
(D) 8 mL

67. Medical control orders the administration of 2 mg of naloxone to an unconscious patient. Naloxone is supplied in a solution concentration of 0.4 mg/mL. How many milliliters should you administer?

(A) 1 mL
(B) 3 mL
(C) 5 mL
(D) 7 mL

68. A physician orders you to administer 0.3 mg of epinephrine 1:1000 solution to an asthmatic. How many milliliters should you administer?

(A) 0.03 mL
(B) 0.3 mL
(C) 3 mL
(D) 30 mL

69. Your unconscious patient requires 100 mg of thiamine prior to the administration of dextrose. Thiamine is supplied 50 mg/mL. How many milliliters should you administer?

(A) 1 mL
(B) 2 mL
(C) 3 mL
(D) 4 mL

70. You must mix a bag of lidocaine to achieve a 4:1 solution concentration. You have a 250-mL bag of solution and a vial of lidocaine that contains 40 mg/mL. How many milligrams of lidocaine should be added to the bag to create a 4:1 concentration?

(A) 500 mg
(B) 1000 mg
(C) 1500 mg
(D) 2000 mg

71. You are ordered to administer a lidocaine drip to a patient. The drip will be administered at 2 mg/min. You add 2 g lidocaine to an IV bag that contains 500 mL of solution. Then you attach a drip set capable of administering 60 gtt/mL. What is your drip rate?

(A) 15 gtt/min
(B) 30 gtt/min
(C) 45 gtt/min
(D) 60 gtt/min

72. You respond to the scene of a 68-year-old female in cardiac arrest. When you hook up the monitor, you see that she is in ventricular fibrillation. After several unsuccessful attempts to defibrillate the patient, the first medication to be administered is epinephrine 1 mg of a 1:10,000 solution. How many milliliters should you administer?

(A) 1 mL
(B) 5 mL
(C) 10 mL
(D) 20 mL

73. A patient has been ordered to receive 300 mL of normal saline solution over the next 2 hours. Using a 500-mL bag of solution and a macro drip set (10 gtt/mL), what drip rate should the Paramedic use in order to achieve this administration?

(A) 20 gtt/min
(B) 25 gtt/min
(C) 30 gtt/min
(D) 35 gtt/min

74. The physician has ordered the patient's infusion in the preceding question increased to 500 mL over the next 2 hours. Using a 500-mL bag of solution and macro drip set (10 gtt/mL), what should you set the drip rate at in order to properly increase the infusion rate?

(A) 40 gtt/min
(B) 42 gtt/min
(C) 44 gtt/min
(D) 46 gtt/min

75. You must administer 1500 mL of normal saline to a patient over a period of 6 hours, using a 1000-mL bag of solution and a 10-gtt/min drip set. How many drops per minute should you administer to deliver this amount?

(A) 38 gtt/min
(B) 40 gtt/min
(C) 42 gtt/min
(D) 44 gtt/min

76. You and your partner are working on an unconscious diabetic. Your partner hands you a syringe and tells you that it contains 100 mg of thiamine in 1 mL of solution. After you push the medication, your partner informs you that he mistakenly filled up the syringe with diphenhydramine. In this situation, what should the Paramedic do?

(A) Ignore the error. The diphenhydramine will probably have no ill effects.
(B) Administer the thiamine and bring the patient to the hospital, making no mention of your error.
(C) Immediately contact medical control and advise them of your error, monitor your patient for ill effects of the medication during transport, document your error, and advise hospital staff on your arrival.
(D) Discuss the situation with your partner after the call, and tell him that you will not cover for him again.

77. You are administering a subcutaneous injection to a patient. Which are the most appropriate needle size and angle of insertion to be used?

(A) 25 gauge and 90 degrees
(B) 18 gauge and 90 degrees
(C) 25 gauge and 45 degrees
(D) 18 gauge and 45 degrees

78. What are the correct needle size and insertion angle for an intramuscular injection?

(A) 21 gauge and 90 degrees
(B) 21 gauge and 45 degrees
(C) 25 gauge and 90 degrees
(D) 25 gauge and 45 degrees

79. You are ordered to administer an endotracheal dose of epinephrine. In administering endotracheal medications, the normal IV dose should be increased. What should the endotracheal dose be if the normal IV dose is 1.0 mg?

(A) 2 to 2.5 mg
(B) 5 to 10 mg
(C) 10 to 15 mg
(D) 15 to 20 mg

80. All of the following drugs are classified as narcotic analgesics EXCEPT

(A) morphine sulfate
(B) meperidine
(C) oxycodone
(D) diazepam

81. A parasympatholytic medication has which of the following effects on the body?

(A) blocks the actions of the parasympathetic nervous system

(B) blocks the actions of the sympathetic nervous system

(C) mimics the actions of the parasympathetic nervous system

(D) mimics the actions of the sympathetic nervous system

82. Atropine sulfate is considered a

(A) parasympathomimetic

(B) parasympatholytic

(C) sympathomimetic

(D) sympatholytic

83. Epinephrine is considered a

(A) parasympathomimetic

(B) parasympatholytic

(C) sympathomimetic

(D) sympatholytic

84. All of the following are beta$_1$ responses EXCEPT

(A) increased force of cardiac contraction

(B) increased bronchodilation

(C) increased heart rate

(D) increased conduction velocity

VENOUS ACCESS AND MEDICATION ADMINISTRATION

ANSWERS

64. **The answer is B.** (Caroline/Little Brown, *Overview of Pharmacology.*) (B) Furosemide (Lasix) is not readily absorbed through the bronchial membranes and therefore is NOT a drug to be administered endotracheally. (A) Lidocaine, (C) epinephrine, and (D) atropine are all easily absorbed through the bronchial membranes. Naloxone and diazepam (Valium) are also easily absorbed and are commonly administered endotracheally. The mnemonic NAVEL will assist the Paramedic in remembering which drugs are absorbed through the bronchial membranes.

65. **The answer is D.** (Caroline/Little Brown, *Overview of Pharmacology.*) (D) You must look at a few variables to arrive at 200 mg. The number before the percent sign (%) denotes how many grams are added to 100 mL (constant) of solution (e.g., 2% indicates that 2 g of drugs is added to 100 mL of solution). Once you have the percent solution broken down into grams, it is easy to figure out the solution concentration of the drug. You have 4 g in 100 mL (4000 mg). Therefore, your solution concentration is 40 mg / 1 mL. Therefore, if you administer 5 mL, you will be administering 200 mg of medication.

66. **The answer is D.** (Caroline/Little Brown, *Overview of Pharmacology.*) (D) In order to complete this calculation, you must transfer the amount of drug into a volume to be administered. If furosemide is supplied 40 mg / 4 mL, then your solution concentration will be 10 mg / 1 mL. Therefore, you will deliver 8 mL for a correct dose of 80 mg.

67. **The answer is C.** (Caroline/Little Brown, *Overview of Pharmacology.*) (C) 5 mL, the correct calculation, would require you to know the desired dose (2 mg) and the dose on hand (0.4 mg/mL). You would divide the dose on hand by the desired dose, in this case 2 mg / (0.4 mg/mL), which would equal 5 mL. (A), (B), and (D) are incorrect.

68. The answer is B. (Brady, *Emergency Pharmacology.*) (B) This calculation is based on the same mathematical formula used in percent solutions. In this instance, a 1:1000 solution equals 1 g in 1000 mL of solution (1000 mg / 1000 mL = 1 mg/mL). Divide the desired dose by the dose on hand, and you arrive at 0.3 mL.

69. The answer is B. (Caroline/Little Brown, *Overview of Pharmacology.*) (B) 2 mL is correct. This calculation uses the formula, desired dose divided by dose on hand. Therefore, the equation is 100 mg / (50 mg/mL) = 2 mL. Answers (A), (C), and (D) are incorrect.

70. The answer is B. (Brady, *Emergency Pharmacology.*) (B) 1000 mg should be added to the 250-mL bag to create a 4:1 concentration. This concentration means that in every 1 mL of solution, you have 4 mg of lidocaine. This is achieved by multiplying the size of your bag of solution by 4 (use 4 because your desired concentration is 4:1). That would equal 1000 mg.

71. The answer is B. (Brady, *Emergency Pharmacology.*) (B) 30 gtt/min. In this situation, you have to determine the amount of lidocaine in the bag per milliliter. If you have a 500-mL bag and have added 2 g of lidocaine, this would make your concentration 4:1. Now that you have the concentration, you must figure out the drip rate. This is done by dividing the desired dose by the dose on hand: (2 mg / min) / (4 mg / mL) = 0.5. Then multiply 0.5 by the rate of the drip set (60 gtt/min) to be used: 0.5 × 60 = 30 gtt/min. (A), (B), and (D) are incorrect.

72. The answer is C. (Caroline/Little Brown, *Overview of Pharmacology.*) (C) Epinephrine 1:10,000 solution (injection) equals 1 g in 10,000 mL of solution. This is equal to 1000 mg/10,000 mL. In order to calculate the number of milliliters needed to deliver 1 mg, you must further break down the concentration to 1 mg/10 mL. If you need to administer 1 mg, then you should administer 10 mL of epinephrine 1:10,000.

73. The answer is B. (Mosby, *Emergency Pharmacology.*) (B) In order to administer volume over time, you must have the following information: volume to be administered, time period of administration, and number of drops per milliliter your infusion set is capable of delivering. To calculate the infusion rate, you must multiply the volume to be administered by the number of drops per milliliter delivered by the solution set (300 × 10 = 3000). Then you must divide that by the time of administration (in minutes, in this case, 120). You should set your drip rate at 25 gtt/min to deliver 300 mL over the next 2 hours.

74. The answer is B. (Mosby, *Emergency Pharmacology.*) (B) Use the following information: volume to be administered, time period of administration, and number of drops per milliliter your infusion set is capable of delivering. Calculate the infusion rate. Multiply the volume to be administered by the number of drops per milliliter delivered by the solution set (500 × 10 = 5000). Then divide that by the time of administration (in minutes, 120). You will set your drip rate at 41.6 gtt/min (rounded to the next highest number, 42) to deliver 500 mL over the next 2 hours.

75. The answer is C. (Mosby, *Emergency Pharmacology.*) (C) Using the formula (volume to be administered times administration set divided by time in minutes of infusion), you should come out with 41.666 gtt/min, which is rounded off to 42 gtt/min. (A), (B), and (D) are incorrect.

76. The answer is C. (Mosby, *Emergency Pharmacology.*) (C) Medication errors may have serious adverse effects on your patient. As a professional, you must immediately report this error to medical control. They may be able to advise you of certain side effects you should look for based on the patient's history. You must closely monitor the patient for adverse reactions and report your error to the receiving hospital. After the call, you must document the error on the run sheet. You should discuss with your partner different ways to avoid this type of event in the future. (A), (B), and (D) are incorrect. You should never ignore a medication error or try to cover up an error with omissions in your report.

77. The answer is C. (Mosby, *Emergency Pharmacology.*) (C) Subcutaneous injections are administered into the subcutaneous tissue, which is relatively superficial. These injections are for small amounts of solution (usually less than 0.5 mL). The proper needle is 23 to 25 gauge and no longer than ⅝ inches. The insertion is done with the bevel up and at a 45-degree angle. (A), (B), and (D) are incorrect.

78. The answer is A. (Mosby, *Emergency Pharmacology.*) (A) The correct needle size for an intramuscular injection is between 19 and 21 gauge and 1 to 1½ inches. The insertion angle is 90 degrees. Intramuscular injections go deep into muscle and therefore require a longer needle. The muscle tissue can usually accommodate up to 5 mL of fluid from an intramuscular injection. (B) and (C) give an incorrect angle and needle size, respectively. (D) gives both an incorrect angle and an incorrect needle size.

79. The answer is A. (Brady, *Emergency Pharmacology.*) (A) Endotracheal medications are absorbed through the pulmonary capillaries by way of bronchial tissue. The normal absorption is almost as fast as IV administration. However, you must increase your dose 2 to 2.5 times the IV dose. In addition, endotracheal medications should be diluted in 10 mL of solution to facilitate absorption. (B), (C), and (D) are incorrect, since the dosages are too high.

80. The answer is D. (Mosby, *Emergency Pharmacology.*) (D) Diazepam (Valium) is classified as a sedative-hypnotic. There are two major groups of sedative-hypnotics: benzodiazepines and barbiturates. Diazepam is a benzodiazepine. (A) Morphine sulfate, (B) meperidine (Demerol), and (C) oxycodone (Percocet or Percodan) are all classified as narcotic analgesic agents.

81. The answer is A. (Mosby, *Emergency Pharmacology.*) (A) A parasympatholytic produces a blocking effect on the parasympathetic nervous system. Parasympatholytics are also known as cholinergic blockers. (B) Sympatholytics (adrenergic blockers) block the actions of the sympathetic nervous system. (C) Parasympathomimetics (cholinergic drugs) mimic the actions of the parasympathetic nervous system. (D) Sympathomimetics (adrenergic drugs) mimic the actions of the sympathetic nervous system.

82. The answer is B. (Mosby, *Emergency Pharmacology.*) (B) Atropine (an anticholinergic) is a parasympatholytic. It acts by blocking the actions of the parasympathetic nervous system by occupying muscarinic receptor sites. (A), (C), and (D) are incorrect.

83. The answer is C. (Mosby, *Emergency Pharmacology.*) (C) Epinephrine is a sympathomimetic (adrenergic drug) that mimics the actions of the sympathetic nervous system. It is considered a nonselective adrenergic drug, which means that it has $beta_1$, $beta_2$, and alpha effects. It increases heart rate and contractility ($beta_1$), as well as vasoconstriction systemically (alpha). (A), (B), and (D) are incorrect.

84. The answer is B. (Mosby, *Emergency Pharmacology.*) (B) Bronchodilation is a $beta_2$ response; the lungs are one of the $beta_2$ effector organs. Other $beta_2$ effector organs include the blood vessels, gastrointestinal tract, and liver. (A) Increased force of cardiac contraction, (C) increased heart rate, and (D) increased conduction velocity are all $beta_1$ effects.

SECTION II:
AIRWAY MANAGEMENT AND VENTILATION

The following topic is covered in Section II:

- Airway and Ventilation

AIRWAY AND VENTILATION

Directions: Each item below contains four suggested responses. Select the **one best** response to each item.

85. The trachea divides into the right and left mainstem bronchi. Which is straighter?

(A) right
(B) left

86. A 54-year-old male is found in severe pulmonary edema. He is sitting bolt upright in a chair, laboring to breathe. You would expect his Po_2 to be

(A) high
(B) low
(C) normal

87. The normal tidal volume for an adult at rest is

(A) 50 mL
(B) 250 mL
(C) 500 mL
(D) 1000 mL

88. A patient has a Pco_2 of 20 mmHg. If his tidal volume is normal, what can you assume about his respiratory rate?

(A) It is normal.
(B) It is slower than normal.
(C) It is faster than normal.
(D) It can be any of the above.

89. Esophageal gastric tube airways should not be used in

(A) unconscious patients
(B) conscious patients
(C) spinal injury patients
(D) patients over 70 years of age

90. When using a MacIntosh laryngoscope blade, the tip of the blade should be placed

(A) between the epiglottis and vocal cords
(B) on the right tonsil
(C) on the uvula
(D) between the epiglottis and the base of the tongue

91. A patient with inspiratory stridor, tracheal tugging, and intercostal retractions is most likely suffering from

  (A) pulmonary edema
  (B) asthma
  (C) chronic obstructive pulmonary disease (COPD)
  (D) upper airway obstruction

92. Absent breath sounds could be an indication of

  (A) pneumothorax
  (B) pneumonia
  (C) severe asthma
  (D) any of the above

93. Air that passes through a narrowed bronchiole produces a sound called

  (A) rales
  (B) rhonchi
  (C) wheezing
  (D) a bronchial sound

94. An increase in respiratory effort when lying flat is known as

  (A) asthma
  (B) orthopnea
  (C) eupnea
  (D) hyperpnea

95. Hyperventilation may be seen in cases of

  (A) anxiety
  (B) pulmonary embolism
  (C) asthma
  (D) any of the above

96. Carbon dioxide is transported in the blood

  (A) in solution
  (B) through interaction with the buffer system
  (C) in combination with hemoglobin
  (D) all of the above

97. All of the following contain dead space EXCEPT

  (A) alveoli
  (B) bronchioles
  (C) pharynx
  (D) trachea

98. Because of the response of hemoglobin to oxygen, which of the following statements is true?

  (A) A P_{O_2} of 60 mmHg produces nearly as much hemoglobin saturation as does a P_{O_2} of 90 mmHg.
  (B) A P_{O_2} of 40 mmHg produces significantly more hemoglobin saturation than does a P_{O_2} of 20 mmHg.
  (C) Both A and B are correct.
  (D) Neither A nor B is correct.

99. Which of the following blood gas values are normal for blood that has completed internal respiration?

  (A) P_{CO_2} 45 mmHg, P_{O_2} 100 mmHg
  (B) P_{CO_2} 40 mmHg, P_{O_2} 100 mmHg
  (C) P_{CO_2} 40 mmHg, P_{O_2} 45 mmHg
  (D) P_{CO_2} 40 mmHg, P_{O_2} 40 mmHg

100. All of the following are components of the alveolar-capillary membrane EXCEPT

  (A) endothelium
  (B) basement membrane
  (C) smooth muscle
  (D) septal cells

101. Surfactant is secreted by the

  (A) goblet cells
  (B) endothelium
  (C) alveolar basement membrane
  (D) septal cells

102. Structure is given to the trachea by

(A) the thyroid cartilage
(B) cartilaginous rings
(C) smooth muscle
(D) basement membrane

103. The bronchioles are composed of

(A) cartilaginous rings
(B) alveolar ducts
(C) smooth muscle
(D) septal cells

Questions 104 to 107 are based on the following scenario.

A 24-year-old woman is complaining of numbness around her mouth, dizziness, and cramps in the extremities. You note that she is breathing very deeply at 32 times per minute.

104. You can assume that her P_{CO_2} is

(A) lower than normal
(B) higher than normal

105. If this is the case, her arterial pH is

(A) higher than normal
(B) lower than normal

106. Thus, she is developing respiratory

(A) acidosis
(B) alkalosis

107. From the situation described above, you can assume that the patient's P_{O_2} is

(A) normal
(B) above normal
(C) below normal
(D) No determination about the P_{O_2} can be inferred from the above information.

108. An oropharyngeal airway may be used to maintain airway in conscious patients.

(A) true
(B) false

109. If a patient is not cyanotic, one can be confident that he is adequately oxygenated.

(A) true
(B) false

110. Confusion and agitation are key signs of

(A) hypoxia
(B) high P_{CO_2}
(C) hyperventilation
(D) all of the above

111. Every patient in respiratory distress should receive oxygen.

(A) true
(B) false

112. The vocal cords lie within the

(A) bronchi
(B) carina
(C) pharynx
(D) larynx

Questions 113 and 114 are based on the following scenario.

You are dining at a restaurant when you notice a man at another table who appears to be in severe distress but is completely silent. He pushes himself away from the table and staggers toward the men's room. You ask him what is wrong but he is unable to speak.

113. The most likely diagnosis in this case is

  (A) acute pulmonary edema
  (B) asthma
  (C) foreign-body airway obstruction
  (D) a heart attack

114. You should immediately

  (A) give him some water to drink
  (B) deliver four back blows
  (C) perform several abdominal thrusts
  (D) do nothing

115. Oxygen and carbon dioxide are exchanged in the lung by

  (A) osmosis
  (B) active transport
  (C) facilitated transport
  (D) diffusion

116. Infants and toddlers are best intubated with which type of laryngoscope blade?

  (A) Miller
  (B) MacIntosh
  (C) curved
  (D) fiber optic

117. The cuff of an endotracheal tube should be inflated with how many milliliters of air?

  (A) 1 to 2 mL
  (B) 5 to 10 mL
  (C) 15 to 20 mL
  (D) 25 to 30 mL

118. The appropriately sized endotracheal tube for a child may be determined by comparing the diameter of the endotracheal tube with the diameter of the child's

  (A) little finger
  (B) thumb
  (C) forefinger
  (D) nares

119. The correct landmark for a cricothyrotomy is

  (A) just above the thyroid cartilage
  (B) just above the cricoid cartilage
  (C) just below the cricoid cartilage
  (D) between the second and third tracheal rings

120. Attempts at intubation should be no longer than how many seconds?

  (A) 5 seconds
  (B) 10 seconds
  (C) 30 seconds
  (D) 60 seconds

121. The appropriate method of measuring an oropharyngeal airway is

  (A) from the nose to the chin
  (B) from the corner of the mouth to the ear lobe
  (C) from the nose to the ear lobe
  (D) from the chin to the ear lobe

122. The narrowest part of the airway of an infant or a toddler is the
(A) thyroid cartilage
(B) cricoid cartilage
(C) oropharynx
(D) nasopharynx

123. The most secure form of airway control is

(A) modified jaw thrust
(B) esophageal gastric tube airway
(C) endotracheal intubation
(D) oropharyngeal airway

124. The primary advantage of nasotracheal intubation is

(A) It may be accomplished more quickly than orotracheal intubation.
(B) It requires no skill at all.
(C) It may be performed without moving the patient's head or neck.
(D) It is easy to perform on a non-breathing patient.

AIRWAY AND VENTILATION

A N S W E R S

85. The answer is A. (Caroline/Little Brown, *The Airway.*) The right mainstem bronchus is straighter and larger as it leaves the carina. As a result, an endotracheal tube that is advanced too far is more likely to be placed in the right mainstem bronchus than in the left.

86. The answer is B. (Caroline/Little Brown, *Breathing.*) Pulmonary edema congests the lungs with excess fluid and interferes with the exchange of oxygen across the alveolar membrane. As a result, the partial pressure of oxygen in the patient's arterial blood falls, leading to hypoxemia.

87. The answer is C. (Mosby, *Airway and Ventilation.*) Although there is variation according to size, the average tidal volume of air exchanged by an adult with each breath at rest is 500 mL.

88. The answer is C. (Mosby, *Airway and Ventilation.*) The partial pressure of carbon dioxide is inversely proportional to the amount of ventilation. As the patient's ventilation increases, the P_{CO_2} falls. The normal P_{CO_2} is 40 mmHg. In order to increase ventilation to achieve a P_{CO_2} of 20 mmHg, the respiratory rate must be increased.

89. The answer is B. (Mosby, *Airway and Ventilation.*) The esophageal gastric tube airway would cause severe gagging and retching in a patient who was conscious and had an intact gag reflex. The esophageal gastric tube airway is also contraindicated for patients who have an increased risk of esophageal damage and bleeding, such as those with corrosive ingestion or preexisting esophageal disease, and for patients less than 60 inches in height.

90. The answer is D. (Brady, *Airway Management and Ventilation.*) The tip of the MacIntosh (curved) laryngoscope blade is placed in the area between the epiglottis and the base of the tongue. This area is known as the vallecula. The tongue is then lifted to provide visualization of the glottic opening. The Miller (straight) laryngoscope blade is placed beneath the epiglottis, and the blade is used to lift the epiglottis directly.

91. The answer is D. (Mosby, *Respiratory Emergencies.*) Inspiratory stridor is created as air passes through a restricted upper airway. As the negative pressure in the lungs cannot be readily equalized, tracheal tugging and intercostal retractions appear. In the case of pulmonary edema, the patient has rapid respirations with rales heard in the chest. In asthma, the chest appears hyperinflated, and wheezes are heard in the chest. COPD patients generally have diminished breath sounds, with some scattered wheezes.

92. The answer is D. (Mosby, *Respiratory Emergencies.*) Breath sounds are created as air moves in and out of the air passages in the lungs. In a pneumothorax, a portion of the lung is collapsed. Breath sounds may not be heard over the area formerly occupied by the collapsed area of the lung. In pneumonia, areas of the lung are filled with fluid and pus. Air may not be able to pass through these areas to produce breath sounds. In severe asthma, the bronchoconstriction may prevent enough air from moving in and out of the lungs to produce breath sounds.

93. The answer is C. (Mosby, *Respiratory Emergencies.*) As air moves through a narrowed bronchiole a high-pitched musical sound known as wheeze is produced. This is most commonly seen in asthmatics. A rale is a fine crackling sound that is most commonly produced by fluid in the alveoli. A rhonchi is a coarser sound produced by fluid and mucous in some of the larger air passages in the lungs. Bronchial sounds are hollow tubular sounds heard near the center of the chest.

94. The answer is B. (Mosby/ACEP, *Glossary.*) Patients with respiratory problems often have increased distress while lying flat. This sign, known as orthopnea, is most commonly seen in patients with pulmonary edema. Asthma is a disease caused by a narrowing of the bronchioles. Eupnea is normal breathing. Hyperpnea is an increase in the depth and rate of respiration.

95. The answer is D. (Caroline/Little Brown, *Breathing.*) Hyperventilation is an increase in the rate and depth of respiration that results in lowered P_{CO_2} levels. It is most commonly associated with anxiety, but hyperventilation may be a response to hypoxia. A pulmonary embolism, for instance, may interfere with the exchange of oxygen. Ventilation is increased in response to the lowered oxygen levels.

96. The answer is D. (Caroline/Little Brown, *Breathing.*) Carbon dioxide is transported through the blood in three ways. Most of the carbon dioxide is present as carbonic acid, which is a product of the bicarbonate buffer system. Some is bound to the hemoglobin in the red blood cells, and a small amount is in solution with the blood plasma.

97. The answer is A. (Mosby, *Airway and Ventilation.*) Dead space consists of areas of the respiratory system where air moves with ventilation but gas exchange does not occur. Gas exchange occurs primarily in the alveoli and to some extent in the alveolar ducts.

98. **The answer is C.** (Brady, *Comprehensive Patient Assessment.*) The affinity of hemoglobin for oxygen begins to level off dramatically after the Pco_2 reaches 50 mmHg. Below this level, small increases in Pco_2 will yield large increases in the percentage of oxygen saturation. The hemoglobin is already nearly completely saturated when the Pco_2 reaches 60 mmHg, and further increases in Pco_2 will yield only small increases in saturation.

99. **The answer is D.** (Mosby, *Airway and Ventilation.*) When arterial blood has completed gas exchange in the alveoli (external respiration), the Po_2 is approximately 100 mmHg, and the Pco_2 is approximately 45 mmHg. After the blood completes its exchange of gases with the cells (internal respiration), the Po_2 has fallen to approximately 40 mmHg, and the Pco_2 has risen to approximately 40 mmHg.

100. **The answer is C.** (Brady, *Airway Management and Ventilation.*) The alveolar capillary membrane consists of a basement membrane to give structure and an endothelial lining across which gas exchange may occur. There are septal cells that secrete surfactant to decrease surface tension and keep the alveoli open. Smooth muscle is found primarily in the bronchioles.

101. **The answer is D.** (Brady, *Airway Management and Ventilation.*) The septal cells of the alveolar capillary membrane secrete surfactant. They are present in the alveolar-capillary membrane, along with the basement membrane and the endothelium. Goblet cells are found in the trachea and other airways.

102. **The answer is B.** (Mosby, *Overview of Human Systems.*) The trachea structure is maintained by a series of cartilaginous rings. These are not complete rings, but are open at the posterior. Without these rings, the trachea would collapse on inspiration. The thyroid cartilage gives shape to the larynx and provides support for the vocal cords. Smooth muscle and a basement membrane are present in the trachea but do not contribute to its structure.

103. **The answer is C.** (Mosby, *Overview of Human Systems.*) The bronchioles are composed primarily of smooth muscle. This allows the bronchioles to open or close in response to respiratory demands. In reactive airway diseases such as asthma, the smooth muscle may cause bronchospasm, which will create a lower airway obstruction. Cartilaginous rings maintain the structure of the trachea. Alveolar ducts connect the alveoli with the respiratory bronchioles. The septal cells are found in the alveolar-capillary membrane and secrete surfactant to keep the alveoli from collapsing.

104. **The answer is A.** (Caroline/Little Brown, *Respiratory Emergencies.*)

105. **The answer is A.** (Caroline/Little Brown, *Respiratory Emergencies.*)

106. **The answer is B.** (Caroline/Little Brown, *Respiratory Emergencies.*)

107. The answer is D. (Caroline/Little Brown, *Respiratory Emergencies.*) This patient is hyperventilating. The rapid and deep respirations will result in increased ventilation. This will cause the arterial carbon dioxide to decrease. A decrease in carbon dioxide will cause the arterial pH to rise and the blood to become more alkaline. This respiratory alkalosis will create a relative hypocalcemia in the tissues. Numbness and spasms of the hands and feet are seen as a result. The rate of respiration and apparent level of carbon dioxide give no indication of the state of oxygenation. A normal patient who hyperventilates would be expected to have a normal or slightly elevated PO_2. Some patients may hyperventilate in response to a decreased PO_2. This is a pitfall in that patients who are hyperventilating are often assumed to have normal oxygenation.

108. The answer is B. (Mosby, *Airway and Ventilation.*) The oropharyngeal airway will cause severe gagging and retching in conscious patients with an intact gag reflex. Alternative methods of airway control, such as manual positioning or a nasopharyngeal airway, should be considered for conscious patients.

109. The answer is B. (Brady, *Airway Management and Ventilation.*) Cyanosis is often a late sign of hypoxia. It may be difficult to detect in patients with dark skin or under dim lighting conditions. Pulse oximetry may be a more sensitive method of determining oxygenation, but it is not one hundred percent reliable. Patients who exhibit signs of respiratory distress should receive high-concentration oxygen regardless of the absence of cyanosis.

110. The answer is A. (Mosby, *General Patient Assessment.*) Patients who are hypoxic tend to be confused and agitated. These patients exhibit significant distress as they struggle to get more oxygen. A high PCO_2 is often seen later in respiratory failure. A high PCO_2 will cause the patient to become lethargic. This is an ominous sign in a patient with respiratory disease.

111. The answer is A. (Caroline/Little Brown, *Breathing.*) Supplemental oxygen should be given to every patient in respiratory distress. Respiratory depression secondary to oxygen drive in COPD patients is a rare phenomenon. Oxygen should never be withheld from a patient with a history of COPD. Sufficient oxygen should be supplied to correct hypoxia, and the patient should be closely monitored for hypoventilation.

112. The answer is D. (Brady, *Anatomy of the Respiratory System.*) The vocal cords are found within the superior opening of the larynx.

113. The answer is C. (Mosby, *Airway and Ventilation.*)

114. The answer is C. (Caroline/Little Brown, *The Airway.*) Patients who develop sudden distress while eating may be the victims of a foreign-body airway obstruction due to food. This condition may easily be mistaken for a heart attack or other medical problem. The term "café coronary" is used to describe patients who have succumbed to an airway obstruction after being misdiagnosed as having a primary cardiac event. The key to diagnosing airway obstruction is the patient's inability to speak. This indicates that no air is able to pass the glottis. In an unresponsive and apneic patient, the inability to ventilate would lead to the diagnosis of airway obstruction. Several abdominal thrusts, also known as Heimlich maneuvers, should be administered to the patient until the obstruction is relieved.

115. The answer is D. (Mosby, *Airway and Ventilation.*) Oxygen moves from an area of high concentration in the alveoli to an area of lower concentration in the blood by the process of diffusion. At the same time, carbon dioxide moves from an area of high concentration in the blood to an area of lower concentration in the alveoli. The specialized alveolar capillary membrane allows this exchange to occur.

116. The answer is A. (Mosby, *Airway and Ventilation.*) Infants and toddlers have a larynx that is more superior and anterior than that of adults. In addition, the epiglottis is larger in proportion to the other structures of the airway. For these reasons, a Miller or straight laryngoscope blade is preferred over a MacIntosh or curved blade. A fiber-optic blade may sometimes deliver a brighter light and may be easier to decontaminate, but it offers no specific advantage for pediatric patients.

117. The answer is B. (Mosby, *Airway and Ventilation.*) Most endotracheal tube cuffs should be inflated with 5 to 10 mL of air. However, there may be a variation due to the difference in interior diameter of the trachea. Inflating with too little air may create an air leak and also allow foreign material to enter the trachea. Too much air and the pressure may damage the inside lining or the trachea. It is best to fill the cuff until significant air leakage just stops.

118. The answer is A. (Caroline/Little Brown, *The Airway.*) An acceptable way of determining the appropriately sized endotracheal tube for a child is to compare the diameter of the tube with the diameter of the child's little finger. Other methods include the use of age-based or length-based charts, and the use of a mathematical formula. Regardless of the method used, there may be a significant difference in the calculated size of the trachea and the actual diameter. For this reason, it is important to have a range of tube sizes immediately available.

119. The answer is B. (Brady, *Airway Management and Ventilation.*) A cricothyrotomy should be performed at the cricothyroid membrane. The membrane lies above the cricoid cartilage and below the thyroid cartilage in the anterior neck.

120. The answer is C. (Brady, *Airway Management and Ventilation.*) Attempts at endotracheal intubation should be limited to 30 seconds. Hypoxia during prolonged intubation attempts is a significant complication of endotracheal intubation. Patients should be hyperventilated prior to intubation attempts in order to optimize oxygenation. Pulse oximetry should be employed when available to monitor the status of the patient's oxygen saturation.

121. **The answer is B.** (Caroline/Little Brown, *The Airway*.) An appropriately sized oropharyngeal airway reaches from the corner of the patient's mouth to the ear lobe. When properly positioned, the flange rests against the teeth.

122. **The answer is B.** (Mosby, *Airway and Ventilation*.) Unlike the adult airway, the airway of an infant or a toddler is more or less funnel shaped, with the narrowest point being at the cricoid membrane. For this reason, endotracheal tubes used for infants and toddlers are not cuffed. A properly sized tube will create its own seal at the narrowest point of the airway.

123. **The answer is C.** (Brady, *Airway Management and Ventilation*.) An endotracheal tube provides the most secure form of airway control. A cuffed endotracheal tube isolates the trachea and prevents the entry of foreign material while assuring that all inspired gas is delivered to the lungs. Manual methods, such as the modified jaw thrust, and simple devices, such as the oropharyngeal airway, cannot prevent the aspiration of gastric contents. The esophageal gastric tube airway will prevent the release of gastric contents but will not protect from blood or other material that may enter the upper airway, and this device is limited to a select group of patients.

124. **The answer is C.** (Brady, *Airway Management and Ventilation*.) Nasotracheal intubation may be performed without moving the patient's head or neck. This makes the technique very useful for trauma patients. It usually takes a longer time to perform nasotracheal intubation because the tube must be advanced carefully through the nose in order to avoid trauma and bleeding. Since this procedure is only performed on patients who are spontaneously breathing, this is not a significant problem. While nasotracheal intubation is a blind procedure, some skill and experience is necessary to ensure success.

SECTION III: PATIENT ASSESSMENT

The following topics are covered in Section III:

- Patient Assessment: History
- Patient Assessment: Physical
- Patient Assessment: Assessment
- Patient Assessment: Communications
- Patient Assessment: Documentation

PATIENT ASSESSMENT: HISTORY

Directions: Each item below contains four suggested responses. Select the **one best** response to each item.

125. The most important source for obtaining information on the patient's history is

(A) witnesses at the scene
(B) the patient's family
(C) the patient
(D) the patient's personal physician

126. Which of the following is an example of an "open-ended" question?

(A) Do you have any allergies?
(B) Have you been hospitalized recently?
(C) Are you under the care of a physician?
(D) What type of pain are you experiencing?

127. The patient's "chief complaint" is described as which of the following components of the medical history?

(A) the reason that the patient has called for assistance
(B) previous episodes of illness
(C) the results of your physical examination
(D) the patient's use of medications

128. All of the following are components of the history of present illness EXCEPT

(A) past medical history
(B) onset of symptoms
(C) quality of pain
(D) severity of pain

129. Your 65-year-old male patient is complaining of severe substernal chest pain radiating to his left arm. He is cool, pale, and diaphoretic. As you begin treatment, your patient tells you that the last time he had this type of pain his doctor told him he had a "bad" heart attack. The information concerning his previous heart attack is part of which component of the patient history?

(A) chief complaint
(B) history of present illness
(C) family history
(D) past medical history

130. Your 42-year-old female patient is complaining of a squeezing chest pain and difficulty breathing. She has no prior history and no other predisposing factors (e.g., smoking). Your evaluation of the patient includes an electrocardiogram, which reveals elevated S-T segments. When asked, the patient informs you that her mother "passed away" at age 47 from a massive heart attack. Her mother's cardiac history is an important piece of information from which component of the medical history?

(A) family history
(B) past medical history
(C) history of present illness
(D) allergies

131. You respond to an elderly patient with an altered mental status. On your arrival, you notice that the apartment is very cold, and you find your patient shivering and exhibiting early signs of hypothermia. Your evaluation of the patient's status based on the living conditions falls into which component of the patient history?

(A) history of present illness
(B) past medical history
(C) chief complaint
(D) social history

132. In questioning your patient with chest pain, he states that he has no difficulty breathing and no nausea. In addition, you notice that he has no jugular venous distention or peripheral edema. These findings should be documented as

(A) pertinent positives
(B) pertinent negatives
(C) symptomatic findings
(D) They should not be documented because they do not offer any clues as to the patient's condition.

133. All of the following are components of the past medical history EXCEPT

(A) patient allergies
(B) medications taken
(C) events preceding the illness or injury
(D) onset of pain

PATIENT ASSESSMENT: HISTORY

A N S W E R S

125. **The answer is C.** (Caroline/Little Brown, *Obtaining the Medical History*.) (C) The patient is always the most qualified person from whom to elicit information. He or she will give you a comprehensive medical history and medication list as well as the symptoms of his or her current illness. (A) Witnesses at the scene can be good providers of information if the patient is unconscious or has suffered injury due to trauma. (B) The patient's family is also an excellent source of patient information when the patient is unable to communicate. (D) The patient's physician will have a wealth of information about the patient, but in emergent situations, the physician may not be readily available to relay the information.

126. **The answer is D.** (Brady, *Patient History*.) (D) When you ask patients about the type of pain they are experiencing, it elicits an explanatory answer. It gives patients a chance to explain how they feel, which, in turn, gives you a greater understanding of their condition. (A), (B), and (C) are all "closed-ended" questions, which generally elicit a yes-or-no response.

127. **The answer is A.** (Mosby, *General Patient Assessment*.) (A) The patient's chief complaint is usually the reason that the EMS system has been activated. It is typically an acute change that affects the patient's normal state. (B), (C), and (D) are also important components of the patient history, but they fall into their own categories in the history.

128. **The answer is A.** (Mosby, *General Patient Assessment*.) (A) The past medical history, although quite an important aspect of the overall patient history, is not a component of the history of present illness. Past medical history is itself a separate component of the overall history. The history of present illness includes (B) onset of symptoms, (C) quality of pain (e.g., squeezing, pressure, or burning), and (D) severity of pain. Other components include radiation of pain as well as aggravating and alleviating factors.

129. The answer is D. (Mosby, *General Patient Assessment.*) (D) The patient's information about his last heart attack falls under past medical history. This piece of information can be significant in your diagnosis. The patient's statement about the last time he had this type of pain should be an indicator that he is suffering from a myocardial infarction. Although this is good information for confirming a diagnosis, the Paramedic should never cease further history taking based on one piece of information. (A), (B), and (C), although important components of the patient's history, are incorrect.

130. The answer is A. (Mosby/ACEP, *Focused and Continued Assessment.*) (A) Family history is an important aspect of the overall patient history. As you see in this case, the patient has no prior medical history. The observation that her mother had a cardiac condition is a critical indicator that she may be suffering from a cardiac-related illness. (B), (C), and (D) are incorrect components of the history in this example.

131. The answer is D. (Mosby/ACEP, *Focused and Continued Assessment.*) (D) The social history may be an important factor in the determination of the patient's illness. Some other examples of social history are smoking, alcohol and drug abuse, employment, and recent travel. These could be all important factors in your diagnosis. Although (A) history of present illness may include the fact that the patient is hypothermic due to living in an unheated residence, that piece of information is obtained from the social history. (B) and (C) are incorrect.

132. The answer is B. (Brady, *Patient History.*) (B) Pertinent negatives are findings that you may expect to be typical of the patient's presentation but that are absent in the patient's complaint. These findings should always be documented on the run sheet. The Paramedic should document all components of the patient history and physical examination, regardless of the fact that they do not support the diagnosis. (A) Pertinent positives are positive findings that support your diagnosis. (C) Symptomatic findings is another term for pertinent positives. (D) is incorrect because all information obtained by the Paramedic should be documented.

133. The answer is D. (Brady, *Patient History.*) (D) Onset of pain is classified in the history of present illness component of the patient history. The onset of pain can be instrumental in the differential diagnosis of certain disease. (A), (B), and (C) are all components of the past medical history. Using the mnemonic AMPLE, the Paramedic can classify the past medical history as follows: A = allergies, M = medications, P = past medical problems, L = last oral intake, E = events preceding the emergency.

PATIENT ASSESSMENT: PHYSICAL

Directions: Each item below contains four suggested responses. Select the **one best** response to each item.

134. All of the following are accepted tools for evaluating airway and breathing in the conscious patient during the primary assessment EXCEPT

(A) inspection
(B) palpation
(C) auscultation
(D) end tidal CO_2 detection

135. All of the following pulse points are generally accepted in the determination of a pulse rate in an adult EXCEPT

(A) brachial
(B) radial
(C) femoral
(D) carotid

136. You are on the scene of a shooting, and your patient is a 43-year-old male who has been shot once in the right upper quadrant of the abdomen. He is hypovolemic during your primary survey. As you assess the skin, you can expect it to appear in any of the following ways EXCEPT

(A) mottled
(B) cyanotic
(C) ashen
(D) jaundiced

137. In the assessment of a patient's mental status using the AVPU scale, the A stands for

(A) alive
(B) alert
(C) appropriate
(D) affect

138. Your patient is a 17-year-old male who has been stabbed in the lower right chest and is complaining of severe difficulty breathing. Examination reveals minor external bleeding, but you note diminished breath sounds on the right side. The right side of the chest is hyporesonant (dull to percussion). This may indicate

(A) tension pneumothorax
(B) pericardial tamponade
(C) hemothorax
(D) subcutaneous emphysema

139. Capillary refill is not a good indicator of hemodynamic status in adults because it can be affected by all of the following factors EXCEPT

(A) hypertension
(B) medications
(C) cold weather
(D) smoking

140. To examine your patient for jugular venous distention, you should elevate the body to what angle?

(A) 15 degrees
(B) 30 degrees
(C) 45 degrees
(D) 60 degrees

141. You are called to a 22-year-old male who is unresponsive upon examination. You find that he has overdosed on an opioid analgesic. You would expect his pupils to be

(A) equal and reactive
(B) constricted
(C) dilated and unresponsive
(D) unequal

142. In auscultating for bowel sounds, you should listen to the patient's abdomen for no less than how many seconds?

(A) 15 seconds
(B) 30 seconds
(C) 45 seconds
(D) 60 seconds

143. Crepitation is best defined as

(A) a yellowish coloration
(B) reddening of an area
(C) a crackling sensation felt on palpation of the skin
(D) a "black and blue"

144. All of the following are techniques for conducting a physical examination EXCEPT

(A) inspection
(B) palpation
(C) percussion
(D) evaluation of mental status

145. You are examining your head-injured patient. As you turn his head, you notice that his eyes move along with the head. This type of response is known as

(A) dysconjugate gaze
(B) raccoon's eyes
(C) anisocoria
(D) doll's-eye response

146. Your 15-year-old female patient is complaining of difficulty breathing from asthma. During your physical examination, you notice that her left pupil is larger than her right pupil. This condition is known as

(A) Battle's sign
(B) dysconjugate gaze
(C) anisocoria
(D) raccoon's eyes

PATIENT ASSESSMENT: PHYSICAL

ANSWERS

134. The answer is D. (Brady, *Patient Assessment.*) (D) End tidal CO_2 detection is used commonly in intubated patients, but it has no value to the Paramedic during the primary assessment, where the determination of a secure airway and breathing is essential. Answers (A) Inspection, (B) Palpation, (C) Auscultation, are all medically accepted practices in the prehospital care arena. These follow the same criteria as look, listen, and feel.

135. The answer is A. (Brady, *Primary Assessment.*) (A) The brachial pulse is the primary pulse point in an infant, but it is not generally used in the assessment of the pulse in an adult. Blood pressure can be estimated by the pulse point. (B) Radial pulses that are present represent a blood pressure above 80 mmHg, (C) femoral pulses represent a blood pressure of approximately 70 mmHg, and (D) carotid pulses generally represent a blood pressure of 60 mmHg.

136. The answer is D. (Brady, *Primary Assessment.*) (D) Jaundice is a condition of increased bilirubin in the blood and is not usually associated with hypovolemic shock. The skin of a patient who is hypovolemic can present as (A) mottled, or blotchy; (B) cyanotic, or blue; or (C) ashen in color. In addition, the patient may present with a pale appearance (pallor).

137. The answer is B. (Mosby/ACEP, *Initial Assessment.*) (B) The AVPU scale is a standard for determination of mental status; it develops a baseline for the patient's overall condition. A = alert or awake, V = voice responsive, P = pain responsive, and U = unconscious or unresponsive. (A), (C), and (D) are incorrect.

138. The answer is C. (Brady, *Head-to-Toe Evaluation.*) (C) Percussion in hemothorax will reveal a chest that is hyporesonant (dull to percussion). This is due to fluid in the chest cavity. In a (A) tension pneumothorax, the chest will be hyperresonant. (B) Pericardial tamponade will not present with abnormal findings during an assessment using percussion, but it will present with muffled heart sounds during auscultation. (D) Subcutaneous emphysema will present with palpable crackling under the skin. This condition is caused by air trapping in the subcutaneous tissues.

139. **The answer is A.** (Brady, *Comprehensive Patient Assessment.*) (B), (C), and (D) are all factors that may cause capillary refill to be delayed and create a false positive in the assessment of the patient with shock. Capillary refill is usually a good indicator in pediatric patients, but it should never be used primarily in the diagnosis of hypoperfusion. Rather, it should be considered a sign of such, and the Paramedic should then identify additional signs and symptoms. (A) Hypertension will not delay capillary refill.

140. **The answer is C.** (Brady, *Head-to-Toe Evaluation.*) (C) To examine the jugular veins for distention, the patient should be placed at a 45-degree angle. Normal jugular venous distention appears in healthy patients while they are supine. The patient who is suffering from right heart failure will present with jugular venous distention even while standing (90-degree angle). (A), (B), and (D) are incorrect.

141. **The answer is B.** (Mosby, *General Patient Assessment.*) (B) The pupils of the patient who has overdosed on an opioid will be constricted. Constricted pupils may also be present in certain patients with head trauma and may sometimes be due to taking certain medications. (A) Equal and reactive is a normal expected response for all patients. (C) Cardiac arrest, central nervous system (CNS) injury, hypoxia, and certain medications may cause dilated and unreactive pupils. (D) Unequal pupils may be caused by CNS injury, eye trauma, and certain eye medications.

142. **The answer is D.** (Caroline/Little Brown, *Physical Assessment.*) (D) In normal patients, you may hear only one or two bowel sounds in a full minute. Therefore, you must listen for that amount of time to properly determine whether the patient does have normal bowel sounds. Patients who have intestinal blockages will have hyperactive bowel sounds. In addition, patients with peritonitis will have hypoactive or no bowel sounds. (A), (B), and (C) are incorrect.

143. **The answer is C.** (Brady, *Comprehensive Patient Assessment.*) (C) Crepitation is a crackling or grating sensation felt on palpation. It is an indicator of subcutaneous emphysema or fracture when the bone ends rub together. (A), (B), and (D) are incorrect.

144. **The answer is D.** (Brady, *Comprehensive Patient Assessment.*) (D) Evaluation of mental status, although part of the primary survey, is not a technique of the physical examination. (A) Inspection, (B) palpation, (C) percussion, and auscultation are the four techniques of the physical examination used by field personnel.

145. The answer is D. (Brady, *Comprehensive Patient Assessment.*) (D) Doll's-eye response is an indicator of head injury. When the head-injured patient's head is moved, the eyes are fixed and move in the direction of the head. The normal response is for the eyes to remain fixed on an object as the head is moved. (A), (B), and (C) are incorrect.

146. The answer is C. (Brady, *Comprehensive Patient Assessment.*) (C) Anisocoria is naturally present in a good percentage of the population. It occurs naturally when one person's pupils are normally different sizes. However, unequal pupils may be a sign of head injury in the trauma patient. (A) Battle's sign is a discoloration over the mastoid process that is indicative of basal skull fracture. (B) Dysconjugate gaze is when the patient's eyes move in different directions, usually from optic nerve damage. (D) Raccoon's eyes are black-and-blue discolorations of the orbits of the eyes, also indicative of basilar skull fracture.

PATIENT ASSESSMENT: ASSESSMENT

Directions: Each item below contains four suggested responses. Select the **one best** response to each item.

147. As an EMS provider, the Paramedic must complete a scene size-up on every call. At what point during the medical or trauma call does the scene size-up begin?

(A) upon arrival at the call
(B) when the Paramedic makes patient contact
(C) when the Paramedic receives the call
(D) when police, fire, or other public-safety officials brief the Paramedic at the scene

148. Identification of potential hazards includes all of the following EXCEPT

(A) surveying the scene for fuel spills
(B) ensuring that a partially collapsed building is properly shored up
(C) identification of the perpetrator of a crime
(D) determination of the presence of carbon monoxide or other agents at a scene with multiple patients complaining of severe headaches and malaise

149. You respond to a motor vehicle accident on a major highway. On your arrival, you see that four cars are involved. What is the importance in the determination of the exact number of patients involved in this accident?

(A) Determining the exact number of patients will assist the Paramedic in requesting additional resources at the scene.

(B) Determining the exact number of patients will assist the Paramedic in knowing how much equipment will be needed.

(C) Determining the exact number of patients will assist the Paramedic in referring patients to the police for reports.

(D) Determining the exact number of patients will assist the Paramedic in billing procedures.

150. Which patient age group would most likely have a fear of strangers, therefore presenting the Paramedic with a difficult patient evaluation?

(A) birth to 6 months
(B) 7 months to 3 years
(C) 4 years to 10 years
(D) adolescents

151. Patients in which age group are most likely to have a fear of disfigurement but can be expected to be fully cooperative with their examination and treatment by a Paramedic?

(A) birth to 6 months
(B) 7 months to 3 years
(C) 4 years to 10 years
(D) adolescents

152. You respond to a 24-year-old female asthmatic. Her breathing is shallow (tidal volume 300 mL), at 28 breaths per minute. What is her minute volume?

(A) 7200 mL
(B) 7400 mL
(C) 8200 mL
(D) 8400 mL

153. You are treating a patient with an altered mental status. He is confused and disoriented. With painful stimuli, he opens his eyes and withdraws from the stimuli. What is his score on the Glasgow coma scale?

(A) 10
(B) 11
(C) 12
(D) 13

154. The respiratory pattern that is characterized by periods of rapid, irregular breaths alternating with periods of apnea is known as

(A) Kussmaul's respirations
(B) eupnea
(C) central neurogenic hyperventilation
(D) Cheyne-Stokes respirations

155. In the assessment of the patient suffering trauma from a motor vehicle accident, which factor will have the most detrimental effect on the patient?

(A) the patient's weight
(B) the type of collision
(C) the speed of the vehicle on impact
(D) the patient's position in the vehicle

156. As part of your ongoing assessment of the unstable trauma patient, you should reassess your patient

(A) every 5 minutes
(B) every 10 minutes
(C) every 15 minutes
(D) every 20 minutes

157. You are assessing an unconscious patient who has snoring respirations. What is the most frequent cause of this type of respiration in the unconscious patient?

(A) blood
(B) vomit
(C) teeth
(D) tongue

158. While assessing your patient's airway, you find that there is a food bolus lodged in the oropharynx. Basic life support maneuvers do not clear the airway. As a Paramedic, what type of intervention should you initially attempt?

(A) abdominal thrusts
(B) needle cricothyroidotomy
(C) direct visualization with laryngoscope and Magill forceps
(D) orotracheal suctioning

159. Your 55-year-old male patient is complaining of difficult breathing. He is cyanotic and breathing 32 times per minute. What is the appropriate oxygen delivery device for this patient?

(A) nasal cannula
(B) bag-valve-mask
(C) nonrebreather mask
(D) blow-by oxygen

160. Your assessment of the trauma patient reveals a patent airway, adequate breathing, but an uncontrolled arterial bleed from the midaxillary artery. Your attempts at bleeding control are unsuccessful. You first priority should be to

(A) Apply direct pressure as well as you can and continue your assessment.
(B) Apply Military Anti-Shock Trousers (MAST pants) to control shock.
(C) Transport immediately, making bleeding control your first priority.
(D) Establish large-bore intravenous access to replace lost blood volume.

161. The average normal pulse range for a newborn is

(A) 120 to 160 beats per minute
(B) 60 to 80 beats per minute
(C) 80 to 120 beats per minute
(D) 80 to 140 beats per minute

162. All of the following are signs of respiratory distress EXCEPT

(A) nasal flaring
(B) tracheal tugging
(C) intercostal retraction
(D) Cheyne-Stokes respirations

163. The Glasgow coma scale uses all of the following variables to identify mental status EXCEPT

(A) respiratory rate
(B) eye opening
(C) motor response
(D) verbal response

PATIENT ASSESSMENT: ASSESSMENT

ANSWERS

147. The answer is C. (Brady, *Scene Size-up.*) (C) The scene size-up begins as soon as the Para-medic is assigned to the call. If Paramedics do a comprehensive review of all the dispatch data, in most cases they will be able to obtain a considerable amount of information, includ-ing scene safety, patient condition, and additional resources responding or needed. (A) Upon arrival at the call, the Paramedic performs the 10-second scene survey. (B) When the Para-medic makes patient contact, the patient history component begins. (D) On-scene briefing by police, fire, or other public-safety officials is also part of the 10-second scene survey.

148. The answer is C. (Brady, *Scene Size-up.*) (C) Identification of perpetrators is the responsi-bility of the police department. Although, as a safety consideration, it is important to know that the perpetrator has left the scene, this responsibility is left to police officers. (A) The Paramedic should survey the scene for fuel spills that could be potentially hazardous to the patient or the Paramedic. (B) Paramedics should never enter a partially collapsed building unless they are specially trained in that type of rescue. The Paramedic should ensure his or her safety by confirming the status of a building prior to entry. (D) Paramedics should try to identify the causative agent at any scene where there are multiple patients complaining of similar symptoms. This will ensure their safety as well as assist in patient care.

149. The answer is A. (Brady, *Scene Size-up.*) (A) As part of the initial scene survey, Para-medics must ensure that they have an accurate patient count in order to request additional resources. This will eliminate any delays in patient care due to lack of personnel. (B), (C), and (D) are incorrect.

150. The answer is B. (Mosby, *General Patient Assessment.*) (B) Children who are 7 months to 3 years old fear strangers and suffer from separation anxiety. These patients have little understanding of their illness and may experience emotional problems associated with their illness or injury. They are best examined and treated in the presence of a parent. (A), (C), and (D) are incorrect.

151. **The answer is D.** (Mosby, *General Patient Assessment.*) (D) Adolescent patients are generally approached as adults, although they have a fear of disfigurement, disability, and death, and the Paramedic should be reassuring and understanding during their care. (A), (B), and (C) reflect incorrect age groups.

152. **The answer is D.** (Caroline/Little Brown, *Breathing.*) (D) To calculate minute volume, you must multiply tidal volume by respiratory rate. In this case, $300 \times 28 = 8400$. This is especially useful in the determination of the patient's oxygenation. The normal tidal volume in an adult is 500 mL, and the normal respiratory rate is 12 to 20 breaths per minute. Therefore, if a patient is breathing at 16 breaths per minute and the tidal volume is 500 mL, the minute volume would be $500 \times 16 = 8000$. (A), (B), and (C) are mathematically incorrect.

153. **The answer is B.** (Caroline/Little Brown, *Injuries to the Head, Neck, and Spine.*) (B) The Glasgow scale is a widely used method of evaluating a patient's level of consciousness. It is scored in three categories: eye opening, motor response, and verbal response, all to outside stimuli. The patient who opens his eyes after painful stimuli is scored a 2 in eye opening. The same patient who withdraws from painful stimuli is scored a 5 in motor response, and the patient who is confused and disoriented is scored a 4 in verbal response. The individual scores are added together to develop a baseline level of consciousness.

154. **The answer is D.** (Caroline/Little Brown, *Physical Assessment.*) (D) Cheyne-Stokes respirations have a variety of neurologic or metabolic causes, some of which are reversible. They are characterized by a respiratory pattern that starts shallow, becomes deeper, and then returns to shallow. This is followed by a period of apnea, and the pattern begins again. (A) Kussmaul's respirations are characterized by rapid, deep respirations presenting in patients with diabetic ketoacidosis. (B) Eupnea is the term for normal breathing. (C) Central neurogenic hyperventilation is characterized by a series of rapid, deep respirations and usually indicates a serious neurologic condition.

155. **The answer is C.** (Mosby/ACEP, *Mechanism of Injury.*) (C) The speed of the vehicle (velocity) creates the most kinetic energy and therefore creates the greatest potential for injury. Although (A) the patient's weight, (B) the type of collision, and (D) the location of the patient in the vehicle are all factors, the single most important factor in any collision is velocity.

156. **The answer is A.** (Brady, *Communication and Documentation.*) (A) The trauma patient should be reassessed often. These patients have rapid changes in vital signs and mental status and should be reevaluated after every intervention. (B), (C), and (D) are incorrect.

157. The answer is D. (Mosby/ACEP, *Assessment of the Critical Patient.*) (D) The tongue is the most frequent cause of snoring respirations in the unconscious patient. The tongue can also cause a complete airway obstruction in patients who cannot control their own airway. The repositioning of the airway may be all that is needed to correct this condition. (A) Blood and (B) vomit usually cause a gurgling sound and are corrected by suctioning. (D) Teeth can cause a total airway obstruction and must also be suctioned out of the airway.

158. The answer is C. (Mosby/ACEP, *Assessment of the Critical Patient.*) (C) The Paramedic should attempt direct visualization with a laryngoscope and Magill forceps to remove the obstruction. (A) Abdominal thrusts in this situation have failed, although that would be one of the first basic life support interventions. (B) Needle cricothyroidotomy should be the last effort made. Needle cricothyroidotomy will provide an airway, but it is not an adequate airway maintenance intervention. (D) Suctioning can be used for smaller obstructions but will not work on a lodged food bolus.

159. The answer is B. (Mosby/ACEP, *Assessment of the Critical Patient.*) (B) The patient with difficulty breathing who has obvious respiratory compromise and a respiratory rate of less than 8 or over 28 should be ventilated using a bag-valve-mask. This will ensure proper tidal volume. (A) The nasal cannula will not deliver an appropriate amount of oxygen to a patient with poor tidal volume. (C) The nonrebreather mask, like the nasal cannula, requires the patient to have acceptable air exchange to properly deliver oxygen. (D) Blow-by oxygen is usually used only with pediatric patients who will not tolerate a mask.

160. The answer is C. (Mosby/ACEP, *Assessment of the Critical Patient.*) (C) Immediate transport is indicated for all patients who have uncontrolled bleeding. There is not time for comprehensive assessments due to the large possibility for fluid loss. (A) The Paramedic should continue to apply direct pressure, but the assessment should not continue, since the priority should be to stop fluid loss. (B) Application of MAST is not indicated for patients with uncontrolled bleeding above the level of the pants. (D) Establishment of a large-bore intravenous access is indicated but is not the first priority. Replacement crystalloid can only replace at a 3:1 ratio to whole blood. Therefore, maintenance of blood volume is the highest priority.

161. The answer is A. (Mosby, *General Patient Assessment.*) (A) The normal pulse rate for an infant is 120 to 160 beats per minute. Infants usually have higher pulse and respiratory rates but lower blood pressures than older children and adults. (B) Sixty to 80 beats per minute is the average pulse rate for an adult. (C) Eighty to 120 beats per minute is the average pulse rate for a 3-year-old child. (D) Eighty to 140 beats per minute is the average pulse rate for a 1-year-old child.

162. The answer is D. (Caroline/Little Brown, *Physical Assessment.*) (D) Cheyne-Stokes respirations are a sign of metabolic or neurological compromise, not of hypoxia or distress.

(A), (B), and (C) are all common signs of respiratory distress. The Paramedic should be aware that the patient might exhibit just one or all of these signs. Additional signs of respiratory distress include tachypnea and anxiety.

163. **The answer is A.** (Brady, *Comprehensive Patient Assessment.*) (B), (C), and (D) are all indicators used for the determination of mental status in patients. The minimum score for all patients is 3, and the maximum score (normal) is 15. (A) Respiratory rate is not measured in the Glasgow coma scale, but it is used as an indicator in the trauma score.

PATIENT ASSESSMENT: COMMUNICATIONS

Directions: Each item below contains four suggested responses. Select the **one best** response to each item.

164. Which of the following transmission modes allows the Paramedic to transmit a patient's electrocardiogram (ECG) while engaging in two-way voice transmission with a telemetry base?

    (A) simplex
    (B) duplex
    (C) triplex
    (D) multiplex

165. When communicating with a telemetry base, the Paramedic should do all of the following EXCEPT

    (A) Monitor the channel to ensure that it is not in use by another crew.
    (B) When speaking, use slang terms to shorten the transmission.
    (C) Repeat all medication orders back to telemetry to ensure the proper medication and dosage.
    (D) Protect the privacy of the patient at all times.

166. All of the following are the responsibility of the EMS dispatcher EXCEPT

    (A) receiving and processing EMS calls
    (B) dispatching and coordinating EMS resources
    (C) coordinating with public-safety agencies
    (D) directing the Paramedic to the appropriate hospital

167. The agency that develops rules and regulations for the use of all radio equipment is

    (A) Federal Communications Commission
    (B) Department of Health
    (C) Department of Transportation
    (D) the individual EMS agency

168. Which of the following are all
EMS–to–medical direction frequencies?

(A) channels 2, 5, 7, and 9
(B) channels 1, 4, 7, and 9
(C) channels 1, 3, 5, and 7
(D) channels 7, 8, 9, and 10

PATIENT ASSESSMENT: COMMUNICATIONS

164. **The answer is D.** (Brady, *EMS Communications*.) (D) Multiplex transmissions allow two-way voice communication at the same time as transmission of an ECG. This feature is highly advantageous to patient care. (A) Simplex transmissions allow only one person to speak at a time, finish his or her transmission, and then receive a response. (B) Duplex communications allow the Paramedic to send and receive voice transmission simultaneously. This is accomplished by the use of dual frequencies. (C) Triplex communications do not exist.

165. **The answer is B.** (Brady, *EMS Communications*.) (B) The Paramedic should never use slang terms while making telemetry contact. These terms are not professionally accepted and may cause confusion as to the patient's actual condition. (A), (C), and (D) are all appropriate techniques for telemetry communication.

166. **The answer is D.** (Mosby, *EMS Communications*.) (D) The EMS dispatcher does not direct the Paramedic to the appropriate hospital. Selecting the hospital is the duty of the Paramedic. (C) In certain circumstances, the EMS dispatcher will coordinate with area hospitals to ensure that no hospitals are overloaded with patients. However, the Paramedic decides where to transport. (A) and (B) are both direct responsibilities of the EMS dispatcher.

167. **The answer is A.** (Mosby, *EMS Communications*.) (A) The Federal Communications Commission (FCC) is responsible for all regulation of radio transmissions and frequency use. The primary functions of the FCC are to license radio frequencies, establish standards for radio equipment, and establish and enforce rules and regulations regarding radio transmissions. (B) The Department of Health, (C) the Department of Transportation, and (D) the individual EMS agency all have roles regarding EMS communications. However, the FCC is the governmental regulatory agency for all EMS agencies.

168. **The answer is C.** (Mosby, *EMS Communications*.) The EMS UHF Special Emergency Radio Services channels consist of 10 EMS radio frequencies. Channels 1 through 8 are all EMS–to–medical direction frequencies. Channels 9 and 10 are dispatch, or steering, channels.

PATIENT ASSESSMENT: DOCUMENTATION

Directions: Each item below contains four suggested responses. Select the **one best** response to each item.

169. The Paramedic should produce a written patient care report on all of the following calls EXCEPT

(A) a trauma call where the patient was transferred to a helicopter crew for transport

(B) a cardiac arrest patient who was pronounced dead at the scene and not transported

(C) an injury patient who refused care and/or transport from the scene

(D) a report of a motor vehicle accident that was discovered to be unfounded on arrival

170. Which of the following data types should be collected on a prehospital care report?

(A) run data, patient data, and treatment data

(B) personal data, patient data, and run data

(C) run data, patient data, and Paramedic personal opinion

(D) patient data, Paramedic personal opinion, and treatment data

171. You respond to the scene of an injury. On your arrival, you find a 29-year-old-male with a laceration to his forehead from falling off a skateboard. After your assessment, you tell the patient that he needs to go to the hospial to get some stitches. The patient refuses, stating he will go to his private physician. What should you document on the patient call report?

(A) nothing, because the patient refused transport

(B) only the patient injury information

(C) only the patient refusal information

(D) all the information from your interaction with the patient

172. During your documentation, you find that you made an error on your patient call report. What is the appropriate method of correcting this error?

(A) Completely cross out the error and write the correct information above it.

(B) Place a line through the error, write the correct information above it, and then initial and date your correction.

(C) Leave the error in place but explain to the emergency department staff that you made an error.

(D) Discard the patient care report and start a new one.

173. The documentation format that follows patient care in the order it was accomplished is known as the

(A) accepted format

(B) chronological format

(C) consumption format

(D) data entry format

PATIENT ASSESSMENT: DOCUMENTATION

ANSWERS

169. **The answer is D.** (Mosby/ACEP, *Communications and Documentation.*) Patient care reports should be completed whenever the Paramedic arrives at the scene and has an interaction with a patient. This report should be completed whether the patient is transported or not. Documentation of (A), (B), and (C) is required by all Paramedics. This documentation serves to provide the EMS agency with a historical chart of patient interaction. (D) An unfounded call is not required to be documented, but some systems require a call report on all EMS calls.

170. **The answer is A.** (Mosby/ACEP, *Communications and Documentation.*) (A) Paramedics should always collect run data, patient data, and treatment data on their call reports. This information has multiple uses and is primarily important in the continuation of patient care in the emergency department. There is no place for a Paramedic's personal opinion on a patient care report. Although the Paramedic's diagnosis is essential to the treatment information, personal opinions should remain off the report. (B), (C), and (D) are incorrect.

171. **The answer is D.** (Mosby/ACEP, *Communications and Documentation.*) (D) Every patient interaction should be documented completely. The Paramedic should obtain all call information and write it on the patient call report. This includes all patients refusing medical care and/or transport. In some cases, the Paramedic should document all attempts to convince the patient to be seen at the hospital. This report should be signed and witnessed at the scene. (A), (B), and (C) are incorrect.

172. **The answer is B.** (Mosby/ACEP, *Communications and Documentation.*) (B) The Paramedic who makes a documentation error can easily correct that error by drawing a line through the erroneous comment and writing the correction above it. This technique will prevent the Paramedic from being falsely accused of trying to cover up his or her error. (A), (C), and (D) are incorrect.

173. **The answer is B.** (Mosby/ACEP, *Communications and Documentation.*) (B) The chronological format follows the care of the patient in the order in which it was done. This is a simple, easy-to-use format in which the Paramedic documents, in time and possible abbreviations, the assessment and care of the patient. This format has the advantage of showing the patient's condition on arrival as well as the response to treatment in real time. This is an important quality-assurance tool to which the Paramedic can refer when legal or call-review issues arise. (A), (C), and (D) are incorrect.

SECTION IV:
PATIENT PRESENTATIONS: TRAUMA

The following topic is covered in Section IV:

- Trauma

TRAUMA

Directions: Each item below contains four suggested responses. Select the **one best** response to each item.

174. Loss of sensation below the nipple line is indicative of a spinal cord injury at the level of

(A) C1
(B) C4
(C) T1
(D) T4

175. The most important sign in evaluating a patient with a head injury is

(A) respiratory pattern
(B) absence of sensation
(C) deep-tendon reflexes
(D) level of consciousness

176. A spinal injury may compromise the function of part of the autonomic nervous system. As a consequence, one would expect to see

(A) bradycardia, due to parasympathetic stimulation
(B) elevated blood pressure, due to vasoconstriction
(C) low blood pressure, due to vasodilation
(D) a rise in body temperature, due to vasoconstriction

177. What changes in vital sign suggest rising intracranial pressure in a head injury patient?

(A) rising pulse rate and rising blood pressure

(B) falling pulse rate and rising blood pressure

(C) falling pulse rate and falling blood pressure

(D) rising pulse rate and falling blood pressure

178. When confronted with a head injury patient who is profoundly hypotensive, your first reaction should be to

(A) intubate and hyperventilate

(B) administer intravenous (IV) dexamethasone

(C) give 2.0 mg naloxone IV

(D) look for signs of other injuries

179. Appropriate management of an unconscious patient with a severe isolated head injury includes all of the following EXCEPT

(A) spinal immobilization

(B) oxygen

(C) close monitoring

(D) rapid infusion of IV fluid

180. After extricating an injured male from a wrecked auto, you observe that he is in respiratory distress. Physical examination reveals an area of his left chest that moves in opposition to the rest of the chest with respiration. The most likely diagnosis is

(A) tension pneumothorax

(B) simple pneumothorax

(C) flail chest

(D) hemothorax

181. Blood in the ear canal of an injured patient must be considered a sign of

(A) ear infection

(B) ruptured eardrum

(C) intracerebral bleeding

(D) skull fracture

182. A 35-year-old male has been dragged unconscious from his burning bedroom by firefighters. The patient is now responsive to pain and has second- and third-degree burns over 40 percent of his body. Your most immediate concern is

(A) preventing infection

(B) controlling airway and ventilation

(C) treating for shock

(D) apply wet dressings to the burns

183. Blistered skin surrounded by a red area best describes

(A) first-degree burn

(B) second-degree burn

(C) third-degree burn

(D) radiation burn

184. An impaled object may be removed if

(A) it is impaled in the eye

(B) it is too large to easily stabilize

(C) it is impaled in the cheek

(D) it interferes with splinting

185. Fractures involving which of the following should not routinely be straightened prior to splinting?

(A) tibia

(B) femur

(C) radius

(D) elbow

186. A properly applied splint must

(A) be twice as long as the fractured bone
(B) be applied very loosely
(C) immobilize the joint proximal and distal to the injured bone
(D) immobilize only the joint proximal to the injured bone

187. The most serious complication of a pelvic fracture is

(A) prolonged disability
(B) urinary incontinence
(C) internal bleeding
(D) urinary tract infection

188. A pulse should always be checked where, in relationship to the fracture site?

(A) proximal
(B) distal
(C) medial
(D) lateral

189. A man was burned on the full circumference of both arms and the full circumference of his right thigh. His percentage of burns is approximately

(A) 18 percent
(B) 27 percent
(C) 32 percent
(D) 36 percent

190. All of following complications of burn injury may require prompt prehospital treatment EXCEPT

(A) shock
(B) airway obstruction
(C) carbon monoxide poisoning
(D) gram-negative sepsis

191. A 25-year-old male has been struck in the right eye with a pool cue. You find a ruptured right globe, an orbital fracture, and no other obvious injury. You should bandage

(A) the right eye tightly
(B) the right eye loosely
(C) both eyes loosely
(D) both eyes tightly

192. Emergency care for most burns caused by chemicals is to treat initially by flooding the affected area with water. Which of the following is an exception to this rule?

(A) hydrochloric acid
(B) dry lime
(C) sodium hydroxide solution
(D) gasoline

193. Which sign should you not specifically attempt to elicit when examining an extremity for signs of a fracture?

(A) crepitus
(B) ecchymosis
(C) swelling
(D) tenderness

194. All of the following are appropriate in treating open fractures EXCEPT

(A) immobilizing the joint above and below
(B) covering the open wound with a sterile dressing
(C) pushing any protruding bone ends back under the skin
(D) checking a distal pulse prior to splinting

195. Which of the following statements about pelvic fractures is true?

(A) No immobilization is necessary.
(B) MAST trousers are contra-indicated.
(C) Injury to the urinary tract is rare.
(D) Patients are usually more comfortable when transported with the knees slightly flexed.

196. Signs of cardiac tamponade include all of the following EXCEPT

(A) muffled heart sounds
(B) tracheal shift
(C) distended neck veins
(D) narrowed pulse pressure

197. The single most important factor in determining the severity of injury in a motor vehicle crash is

(A) the speed of impact
(B) the size of the auto involved
(C) the weight of the victim
(D) the direction of impact

198. The second collision in a motor vehicle crash occurs when

(A) the vehicle collides with another object
(B) the interior of the vehicle collides with the exterior
(C) the occupants collide with the interior of the vehicle
(D) the organs collide with the interior of the occupants

199. Aortic rupture is a major cause of death in which type of motor vehicle collision?

(A) frontal impact
(B) rollover
(C) rear impact
(D) side impact

200. Fractures of the calcanei and lumbar spine are most commonly seen as a result of

(A) high-speed motor vehicle collisions
(B) falls from a height of greater than 15 feet
(C) motor vehicle–pedestrian accidents
(D) bicycle accidents

201. Which of the following is most vulnerable to primary blast injury from the pressure wave of an explosion?

(A) heart
(B) liver
(C) lungs
(D) long bones

202. The wound area of tissue damage from a medium-velocity handgun bullet will usually be

(A) the same as the diameter of the bullet
(B) one-half the diameter of the bullet
(C) twice the diameter of the bullet
(D) 20 times the diameter of the bullet

203. The presence of a clearly palpable radial pulse suggests a systolic blood pressure of at least

(A) 60 mmHg
(B) 80 mmHg
(C) 100 mmHg
(D) 120 mmHg

204. Normal capillary refill is

(A) less than 1 second
(B) less than 2 seconds
(C) greater than 2 seconds
(D) 2 to 4 seconds

205. Crepitus felt over a large area of the chest is a sign of

(A) hemothorax
(B) subcutaneous emphysema
(C) cardiac contusion
(D) aortic rupture

206. Which of the following statements is true regarding the use of bag-valve-mask to ventilate victims of multiple trauma?

(A) It rarely provides effective ventilation.
(B) It cannot be used in cases of thoracic trauma.
(C) It may require two persons to utilize effectively.
(D) It does not increase the danger of tension pneumothorax.

207. Referred pain to the left shoulder is often seen in cases of

(A) lacerations of the liver
(B) right hemothorax
(C) fracture of C_1
(D) ruptured spleen

208. Distended neck veins in a trauma patient are most likely a sign of

(A) cervical spine injury
(B) hemothorax
(C) tension pneumothorax
(D) profound shock

209. The preferred manual method of maintaining an airway in a trauma patient is

(A) modified jaw thrust
(B) head tilt, chin lift
(C) head tilt, neck lift
(D) triple airway maneuver

210. In cases of tension pneumothorax, the trachea will shift

(A) toward the injured side
(B) toward the uninjured side
(C) anteriorly in the neck
(D) posteriorly in the neck

211. Premature ventricular contractions caused by a cardiac contusion should be treated with

(A) rapid infusion of IV fluid
(B) MAST
(C) hyperventilation
(D) IV lidocaine

212. Severe cases of flail chest should be treated with

(A) positive-pressure ventilation
(B) cricothyrotomy
(C) manual stabilization
(D) needle decompression

213. A patient who opens his eyes to verbal stimulation, is disoriented, and localizes pain has a Glasgow coma scale rating of

(A) 13
(B) 12
(C) 11
(D) 10

214. Which of the following may be easily mistaken for an acute myocardial infarction?

(A) pulmonary contusion
(B) pericardial tamponade
(C) aortic rupture
(D) cardiac contusion

215. Ideally, the time spent on the scene with a critical trauma patient should be

(A) less than 10 minutes
(B) more than 10 minutes
(C) less than 20 minutes
(D) as long as necessary to assess and treat every injury

216. The most significant factor in determining the amount of kinetic energy is

(A) mass
(B) velocity
(C) sectional density
(D) angular momentum

217. Tenderness, guarding, rigidity, and distention of the abdomen are signs of

(A) injury to the superficial abdominal muscles
(B) anxiety
(C) injury to internal abdominal organs
(D) shock

218. If you have a patient who presents with dyspnea, hoarseness, and facial burns after being trapped in a confined space with a fire, you should consider

(A) IV fluid replacement
(B) giving copious amounts of water by mouth
(C) endotracheal intubation
(D) sedation with diazepam

219. Which of the following statements is not true about electrical burns?

(A) There is a danger of cardiac dysrhythmia.
(B) They are usually only superficial.
(C) There may be an exit wound.
(D) There may be deep-tissue damage far from the site of the surface injury.

220. In high-velocity gunshot wounds, the exit wound is

(A) the same diameter as the entrance
(B) round with a clearly defined edge
(C) smaller than the entrance due to bullet fragmentation
(D) larger than the entrance and irregularly shaped

221. The preferred method of controlling severe bleeding is

(A) direct pressure
(B) vascular clamps
(C) tourniquet
(D) elevation

222. The greatest danger in facial injuries is

(A) hypovolemic shock
(B) disfigurement
(C) airway compromise
(D) severe pain

223. Which of the following is least useful in treating hypovolemic shock?

(A) MAST
(B) IV volume replacement
(C) bleeding control
(D) vasopressors

224. What is the best clue for determining the possible injuries that a patient may have sustained in a crash?

(A) mechanism of injury
(B) debris
(C) condition or injuries of the other occupants
(D) length of skid marks

225. How much of the "golden hour" is given to the prehospital medical care provider for scene assessment and care?

(A) 1 minute
(B) 10 minutes
(C) 20 minutes
(D) 30 minutes

226. The decision of whether to transport a patient immediately or to attempt on-scene care is one of the most critical decisions you will make during a medical emergency.

(A) true
(B) false

227. As you double the speed of an object, its ability to cause trauma is

(A) reduced by one-half
(B) unchanged
(C) doubled
(D) quadrupled

228. Blunt trauma has little effect on internal organs because the wound does not penetrate the skin.

(A) true
(B) false

229. The anatomical region most commonly injured in the rear-end impact is the

(A) head
(B) neck
(C) chest
(D) extremities

230. The hollow-point, soft-tipped bullet is designed to increase the profile and thereby the rate of energy exchanged.

(A) true
(B) false

231. Generally, powder burns and tattooing around the entrance wound suggest

(A) a gun used at close range
(B) a high-powered rifle
(C) use of a black powder
(D) use of a "dum-dum" bullet

232. The major reason for allowing fluid to drain from the nose or ear is that

(A) It may release intracranial pressure.
(B) Its flow will prevent pathogens from entering the meninges.
(C) It is impossible to stop the flow anyway.
(D) Regeneration of cerebrospinal fluid is beneficial to the healing process.

233. The injury that damages the brain on the side opposite of the impact is called

(A) subdural hematoma
(B) epidural hematoma
(C) contrecoup
(D) a concussion

234. The collection of blood in front of a patient's pupil and iris due to trauma is known as

(A) hyphema
(B) glaucoma
(C) retinopathy
(D) hematoma

235. For a patient with a possible spine injury, manual stabilization should be maintained until

(A) a cervical collar is applied
(B) the patient begins to object
(C) the patient has no pain
(D) the patient is immobilized with a spine board

236. Prolonged intubation attempts may cause dysrhythmias and increased intracranial pressure in the head injury patient.

(A) true
(B) false

237. Hyperventilating a head injury patient at 20 breaths per minute

(A) lowers Pa_{CO_2}, decreasing cerebral blood flow
(B) lowers Pa_{O_2}, decreasing cerebral blood flow
(C) increases Pa_{CO_2}, increasing cerebral blood flow
(D) increases Pa_{O_2}, increasing cerebral blood flow

238. What is the best way to control severe arterial bleeding from the neck?

(A) careful direct pressure
(B) tourniquet
(C) pressure dressing with tight bandage
(D) an occlusive dressing covered with a dressing

239. A patient with a head injury should be observed for hypothermia or hyperthermia.

(A) true
(B) false

240. A foreign body impaled in the eye should be managed with

(A) a tight dressing over the eye
(B) a protective cup over the eye
(C) removal of the object and bandaging of the eye
(D) a loose dressing over the object

241. The area between the visceral and parietal pleura is

(A) filled with air
(B) a potential space
(C) filled with fluid
(D) part of the diaphragm

242. Pain in the right flank and bloody urine after a motor vehicle crash would lead you to suspect injury to

(A) kidney
(B) liver
(C) spleen
(D) heart

243. A stab wound located at the margin of the lower ribs on the anterior of the body should be suspected of causing injury to

(A) abdominal organs only
(B) thoracic organs only
(C) abdominal and thoracic organs
(D) the spine

244. Rib fractures are not routinely immobilized because to do so might

(A) cause severe pain
(B) cause a flail chest
(C) increase the chances of atelectasis and pneumonia
(D) increase bleeding into the chest

245. A flail segment of the chest

(A) moves in the opposite direction of the rib cage during respiration
(B) moves along with the ribcage during respiration
(C) will not move during respiration
(D) moves when the patient is not breathing

246. Frothy blood bubbling from a chest wound is a sign of

(A) flail chest
(B) hemothorax
(C) open pneumothorax
(D) tension pneumothorax

247. A male patient fell from a ladder, striking his chest on some building materials. The patient initially complained of pleuritic pain on the right side of his chest, and some crepitus could be felt over the third and fourth ribs on the right side. En route to the hospital, the patient developed severe shortness of breath and signs of shock. You should suspect

(A) tension pneumothorax
(B) ruptured aorta
(C) intraabdominal bleeding
(D) traumatic asphyxia

248. A collection of blood in the sac around the heart may cause

(A) myocardial infarction
(B) pericardial tamponade
(C) cardiomyopathy
(D) congestive heart failure

249. All of the following are signs of pericardial tamponade EXCEPT

(A) rapid thready pulse
(B) narrowing pulse pressure
(C) jugular vein distention
(D) tracheal deviation

250. In the absence of a spinal injury, a patient with a chest injury is best transported

(A) lying on the uninjured side
(B) lying on the injured side
(C) in the Trendelenburg position
(D) lying on the left side

251. The correct location for pleural decompression is

(A) second intercostal space, mid-clavicular
(B) third intercostal space, midaxillary
(C) fifth intercostal space, mid-clavicular
(D) fifth intercostal space, immediately adjacent to the sternum

252. You have placed an air-occlusive dressing over a stab wound to the chest. Within a few minutes, the patient begins to have severe difficulty in breathing. Your first action is

(A) Intubate and hyperventilate the patient.
(B) Roll the patient onto the uninjured side.
(C) Unseal the wound.
(D) Increase the percentage of oxygen given to the patient.

253. A myocardial contusion is treated the same as

(A) tension pneumothorax
(B) pericardial tamponade
(C) flail chest
(D) myocardial infarction

254. A male patient has been stabbed in the chest. The knife is still protruding from the patient's anterior chest. The patient complains of pain upon inspiration. You should

(A) Stabilize the knife in place with bulky dressings.
(B) Remove the knife and leave the wound open to the air.
(C) Remove the knife and place an airtight dressing over the wound.
(D) Perform a needle decompression of the chest.

255. An abdominal wound with a loop of bowel protruding through it should be managed by

(A) leaving it exposed to the air
(B) covering with a dry sterile dressing
(C) replacing the bowel carefully back through the wound
(D) covering with a moist sterile dressing

256. A soft-tissue injury that results when a joint is moved beyond its normal range of motion is known as a

(A) strain
(B) sprain
(C) dislocation
(D) contusion

257. A suspected dislocation should be managed

(A) by immobilizing the bone above the joint only
(B) by immobilizing the bone below the joint only
(C) by immobilizing the bones above and below the joint
(D) without immobilization

258. Which of the following fractures is most likely to cause life-threatening hemorrhage?

(A) humerus
(B) clavicle
(C) tibia
(D) femur

259. The greatest danger of a fractured pelvis is

(A) severe hemorrhage
(B) permanent deformity
(C) injury to the bladder
(D) paralysis

260. Prior to splinting a fractured elbow, you detected a strong distal pulse and the patient had normal motion and sensation. After splinting, you are unable to feel a distal pulse and the patient complains of numbness in his fingers. You should first

(A) Remove the splint and reapply it.
(B) Remove the splint and do not attempt to reapply it.
(C) Loosen the splint and recheck the pulse.
(D) Transport the patient to the hospital.

261. While attempting to realign an angulated fracture, you meet resistance and the patient complains of extreme pain. You should

(A) Apply more force to the limb.
(B) Rotate the limb slowly while applying force.
(C) Apply a traction splint.
(D) Splint the fracture in its present position.

262. Dislocations should routinely be splinted

(A) after being realigned
(B) as they are found
(C) in an extended position
(D) in a flexed position

263. The most effective device for splinting a fractured femur is

(A) a traction splint
(B) a PASG
(C) an air splint
(D) a rigid board splint

264. Pillow splints may be used for

(A) fracture of femur
(B) knee fractures
(C) humerus fractures
(D) ankle fractures

265. A collection of blood under the skin is

(A) a hematoma
(B) a contusion
(C) a laceration
(D) an abrasion

266. A wound that is susceptible to infection with tetanus and other anaerobic bacteria is

(A) incision
(B) puncture
(C) contusion
(D) avulsion

267. An injury where soft tissue has been torn away is known as

(A) a contusion
(B) an avulsion
(C) an abrasion
(D) an amputation

268. A type of open wound with jagged edges caused by tearing forces is known as

(A) a laceration
(B) an incision
(C) an abrasion
(D) a puncture

269. Patients who have been trapped in an enclosed space with a combustion will most likely suffer from

(A) cyanide poisoning
(B) thermal burns
(C) heat stroke
(D) carbon monoxide poisoning

270. Third-degree burns may be distinguished from first- and second-degree burns by

(A) lack of pain
(B) lack of blistering
(C) color
(D) oozing of fluid

271. Which of the following burns is the most serious?

(A) second-degree burns to the entire left arm
(B) third-degree burns to the right lower leg
(C) first-degree burns to the entire body
(D) second-degree burns around the mouth and nose

272. Which pressure point may be used to control severe bleeding from the area of the wrist?

(A) femoral
(B) temporal
(C) brachial
(D) popliteal

273. Which IV fluid solution should be used for burn patients?

(A) D_5W
(B) normal saline solution
(C) ½ normal saline solution
(D) Ringer's lactate

274. The immediate management for most chemical burn injuries is

(A) a dry, sterile dressing
(B) irrigation with alcohol
(C) irrigation with copious amounts of water
(D) applying a neutralizing agent

275. Skin contaminated with phenol should be initially irrigated with which of the following?

(A) water
(B) soap water
(C) alcohol
(D) mineral oil

276. How should contamination and burns from dry lime be managed?

(A) Irrigate with alcohol.
(B) Brush the chemical away and then irrigate with water.
(C) Apply a baking soda solution.
(D) Irrigate with water immediately.

277. Which of the following would NOT lead you to suspect a spinal injury?

(A) a spider crack in the windshield
(B) a large contusion on the forehead
(C) numbness and tingling in the extremities
(D) a rapid pulse

278. Which of the following would NOT be a reason for immediate transport to a trauma center?

(A) suspected lumbar spine injury
(B) signs of shock
(C) unstable pelvic fracture
(D) deteriorating level of consciousness

279. A tourniquet should always be used to control bleeding from an amputation.

(A) true
(B) false

280. Priapism is seen in cases of

(A) cardiac tamponade
(B) airway obstruction
(C) hypovolemia
(D) spinal injury

281. If a patient's body will not conform to the shape of the backboard, leaving large voids and making it difficult to stabilize the patient, you should

(A) not use a backboard and transport on the ambulance cot
(B) use noncompressible padding to fill the void
(C) use a short board
(D) force the patient down to the board

282. Sandbags are not used to stabilize the head of a spinal injury patient because

(A) Sandbags cannot hold the patient's head securely.
(B) Sandbags are very expensive.
(C) The patient's head may be pushed to the side by the weight of the bags.
(D) Sandbags are very difficult to use.

283. A 7-year-old patient has fallen from a piece of playground equipment. Upon your arrival, you find that the child is not responsive to voice or pain and has slow, snoring respirations. Your most immediate action would be to

(A) Perform endotracheal intubation while maintaining in-line stabilization.
(B) Maintain in-line stabilization and open the airway with a jaw thrust.
(C) Open the airway using the head tilt, chin lift.
(D) Insert an esophageal obturator airway and ventilate with a bag-valve-mask.

284. Before extricating a patient from an automobile crash, you should check motor and sensory function in all extremities and document your findings.

(A) true
(B) false

285. A 43-year-old man was the driver in a motor vehicle crash. Examination of the patient reveals a laceration on the forehead, bruising of the chest, and a tender abdomen. The patient was the unrestrained driver of a compact car that was struck head-on by a pickup truck. The patient is responsive to voice but is disoriented. His blood pressure is 80/50, pulse 125, and respiratory rate 16. Neck veins are flat, and breath sounds are equal bilaterally. The patient's skin is pale, cool, and diaphoretic. The patient's hypotension is most likely due to

(A) hypoxia
(B) hypovolemia
(C) a tension pneumothorax
(D) pericardial tamponade

286. A 25-year-old male was struck by an auto. His right thigh is painful. Physical examination reveals tenderness in the thigh and bruising. There is also shortening and external rotation of the right leg. The most appropriate splint would be

(A) a pillow splint
(B) a traction splint
(C) a sling and swathe
(D) splinting of the uninjured leg

287. The most frequently fractured facial bone is the

(A) nose
(B) maxilla
(C) zygoma
(D) mandible

288. The victim of a motor vehicle accident appears to be in severe distress. The patient has stridorous respirations, and subcutaneous air can be felt in the anterior neck. Which of the following is the most likely cause of this patient's presentation?

(A) zygoma fracture
(B) fractured larynx
(C) aortic disruption
(D) simple pneumothorax

289. The bone that composes the lower third of the face is the

(A) ethmoid
(B) mandible
(C) maxilla
(D) zygoma

290. Increased intracranial pressure may cause

(A) tachycardia
(B) hypotension
(C) abnormal breathing patterns
(D) increased alertness

291. Bilateral periorbital ecchymosis is also referred to as

(A) Battle's sign
(B) Cullen's sign
(C) raccoon's eyes
(D) McBurney's sign

292. Which of the following is true about Glasgow coma scale?

   (A) A score of 3 is normal.
   (B) A score of 7 represents coma.
   (C) A score of 12 accompanies brain death.
   (D) A score of 15 is indicative of a poor prognosis.

293. An injured hand should be immobilized

   (A) flat on a board splint
   (B) with a pillow
   (C) in the position of function
   (D) to the other hand

294. The mechanism of injury associated with striking the head against the windshield of an automobile is

   (A) distraction
   (B) whiplash
   (C) axial loading
   (D) hyperflexion

295. A possible complication of a parietal or temporal skull fracture is

   (A) epidural hematoma
   (B) intraventricular hematoma
   (C) subdural hematoma
   (D) subarachnoid hemorrhage

296. Signs of hypovolemic shock include

   (A) pale skin, tachycardia, and hypotension
   (B) dilated pupils, pale skin, and bounding pulse
   (C) dilated pupils, bradycardia, and flushed skin
   (D) bounding pulse, flushed skin, and bradycardia

297. Pregnant patients near term who have suffered significant trauma should be transported

   (A) lying supine
   (B) lying in the left lateral recumbent position
   (C) in the Trendelenburg position
   (D) in the semi-Fowler's position

298. Trauma patients should have

   (A) a saline lock
   (B) one IV with a small-bore catheter
   (C) one IV with a large-bore catheter
   (D) two IVs with large-bore catheters

TRAUMA

ANSWERS

174. The answer is D. (Mosby/ACEP, *Orthopedic Injuries*.) An injury to the spinal cord at the level of the fourth thoracic vertebra will cause a loss of sensation and motor ability below the nipple line. Injuries at C1 and C4 will cause quadriplegia and will interfere with normal respirations. Injuries at T1 will cause a loss of function below the shoulders.

175. The answer is D. (Mosby/ACEP, *HEENT Trauma*.) An alteration in the level of consciousness is the most important sign when evaluating a patient with a head injury. A deteriorating mental state is an early sign of increasing intracranial pressure, seen in serious head injury. Alteration in respiratory patterns is often a very late sign of a serious head injury. Loss of sensation and abnormal deep-tendon reflexes are difficult to continually assess and may be to due to a spinal or local injury.

176. The answer is C. (Brady, *Head, Neck and Spine Injury*.) Injury to the sympathetic nervous system may accompany injury to the spine. Dysfunction of the sympathetic nervous system will cause vasodilation and subsequent fall in blood pressure. There is not normally any parasympathetic stimulation; therefore, bradycardia would not be present, but the dysfunction of the sympathetic nervous system would prevent tachycardia in compensation for the fall in blood pressure. The vasodilation will cause a fall in body temperature.

177. The answer is B. (Mosby/ACEP, *HEENT Trauma*.) Rising blood pressure and falling pulse rate seen in serious head injuries is known as Cushing's reflex. As a response to the decreased cerebral perfusion caused by rising intracranial pressure, the systolic blood pressure will rise. High systolic blood pressure will activate receptors in the carotid bodies, resulting in bradycardia.

178. The answer is D. (Caroline/Little Brown, *Injuries to the Head, Neck, and Spine.*) Isolated head injuries will rarely cause hypotension. The patient should be examined for other injuries that may be sources of bleeding. Any external bleeding should be controlled, and signs of internal bleeding should be managed with rapid transport and IV fluid replacement. Intubation and hyperventilation are used to treat rising intracranial pressure, which will cause hypertension. Dexamethasone and naloxone will have no effect on traumatic hypotension.

179. The answer is D. (Mosby/ACEP, *HEENT Trauma.*) A rapid infusion of IV fluids may cause an increase in intracranial pressure in a patient with a head injury. Intravenous fluids should be kept at a KVO rate unless the patient becomes hypotensive. In that case, IV fluids should be administered to restore normal blood pressure. Spinal immobilization, oxygen, and close monitoring are appropriate for the management of severe head injury.

180. The answer is C. (Mosby/ACEP, *Truncal Trauma.*) An area of the chest moving in opposition to the rest of the chest, known as paradoxical respiration, is seen when multiple rib fractures disrupt the integrity of the chest wall. This condition is known as flail chest. Dyspnea and decreased breath sounds are signs of pneumothorax and hemothorax. Distended neck veins, difficult ventilation, and tracheal deviation are signs of tension pneumothorax.

181. The answer is D. (Mosby, *Trauma.*) A basal skull fracture may cause leakage of blood and cerebrospinal fluid from the ears. A ruptured eardrum or infection may also cause blood in the ear canal, but a skull fracture must be considered until it can be ruled out. Intracerebral bleeding will not enter the ear canal unless there is accompanying skull fracture.

182. The answer is B. (Mosby/ACEP, *Burn Injuries.*) Patients suffering severe burn injury in an enclosed area are likely to have burns to the airway and respiratory tract. Airway obstruction due to edema and respiratory difficulty may develop rapidly. These must be managed immediately. Shock from burns is not likely to occur rapidly in the field, and infections are not seen in the prehospital phase. Burn dressings should be delayed until the airway is secure, and patients with extensive burns should have dry, sterile dressings.

183. The answer is B. (Caroline/Little Brown, *Wounds and Burns.*) Second-degree burns, also known as partial-thickness burns, are characterized by blisters surrounded by reddened skin. First-degree burns, also known as superficial burns, are characterized by reddened, painful skin. Third-degree burns, also known as full-thickness burns, are characterized by dry, painless charred or brown or white skin. Radiation is a form of energy that may cause any degree of burn.

184. The answer is C. (Brady, *Head, Neck and Spine Injury.*) Impaled objects in the cheek should be removed because they may cause airway obstruction. The end of the object should be located, and the object should be gently removed the way that it entered. Objects impaled in the eye should be stabilized in place and the other eye loosely bandaged. Large objects should be cut so they can be stabilized.

185. The answer is D. (Mosby, *Trauma.*) Fractures involving joints should be splinted in place unless there are signs of neurovascular compromise. In that case, one attempt at realigning the joint may be attempted. Long-bone fractures should be gently realigned prior to splinting.

186. The answer is C. (Caroline/Little Brown, *Fractures, Dislocations, and Sprains.*) In order to properly stabilize a long-bone fracture, a splint should include both joints that are adjacent to the affected bone. A splint should be applied so as to prevent unnecessary movement, but not be too snug as to affect nerve or circulatory function.

187. The answer is C. (Mosby/ACEP, *Orthopedic Injuries.*) Severe internal bleeding is the most serious complication of pelvic fracture. Unstable pelvic fractures may affect many blood vessels and supply a large area for blood to collect. Prolonged disability and urinary tract problems are complications, but they are not normally life threatening.

188. The answer is B. (Mosby/ACEP, *Orthopedic Injuries.*) Prior to any treatment, a pulse should be assessed distal to all fractures. Vascular compromise is a complication of fracture. Distal pulses should also be checked after splinting. If a pulse is lost after splinting, the splint should be adjusted to allow for the return of circulatory function.

189. The answer is B. (Mosby/ACEP, *Burn Injuries.*) Using the standard adult rule of nines, each arm is 9 percent and the thigh is also 9 percent, for a total of 27 percent.

190. The answer is D. (Caroline/Little Brown, *Wounds and Burns.*) Infection is a late complication of burn injury that occurs during the in-hospital phase of treatment. Infections are managed with topical and systemic antibiotics that are not available to prehospital providers. Airway obstruction is the most immediate complication of burn injury that must be managed in the field. Carbon monoxide poisoning is commonly seen in burn patients, and it should be managed with high-concentration oxygen. Shock is not common in the prehospital phase but should be treated with IV fluids.

191. The answer is C. (Mosby/ACEP, *HEENT Trauma.*) In cases of eye injuries, both eyes should be bandaged. This will minimize movement of the injured eye. Bandages should be applied loosely so as to prevent further damage to the eye.

192. The answer is B. (Caroline/Little Brown, *Wounds and Burns.*) Dry corrosive powders, such as lime, should be brushed away first before flooding the area with copious amounts of water. Applying water to large amounts of dry corrosive material may spread the chemical and cause further injury. Liquid corrosives should be treated initially by irrigation with water.

193. The answer is A. (Caroline/Little Brown, *Fractures, Dislocations, and Sprains.*) Crepitus is the sound or sensation that is observed when broken bone ends move against each other. While this may occur incidentally during physical examination, it is accompanied by pain and should never be intentionally caused. Ecchymosis, swelling, and tenderness are observed passively, and are not caused by the examination.

194. The answer is C. (Mosby, *Trauma.*) No attempt should be made to push protruding bone ends back into place. To do so may cause damage to surrounding structures. Checking distal circulation, covering wounds with sterile dressings, and immobilizing both joints adjacent to the fractured bone are all appropriate treatment.

195. The answer is D. (Mosby/ACEP, *Orthopedic Injuries.*) Most patients with pelvic fractures will be more comfortable if transported with their knees slightly flexed. This will allow the pelvis to be better supported on the spine board. Patients with a pelvic fracture should be immobilized to ease transportation and prevent further injury. MAST trousers may be used to treat hypotension secondary to unstable pelvic fracture. Patients with pelvic fracture commonly have injury to the urinary bladder and urethra.

196. The answer is B. (Caroline/Little Brown, *Chest Injuries.*) Tracheal shift is a sign that is seen in tension pneumothorax when the lung is pushed away from the affected side. Muffled heart sounds, distended neck veins, and narrowed pulse pressure are classical signs of cardiac tamponade known as Beck's triad.

197. The answer is A. (Brady, *The Kinetics of Trauma.*) The amount of energy released in a collision is what determines the severity of injury. The energy of objects in motion is calculated by the equation $E = mv^2$. The velocity (v) is the most significant factor in determining energy. The mass and size of the vehicles and victims has a lesser effect on the amount of energy released.

198. The answer is C. (Brady, *The Kinetics of Trauma.*) The typical motor vehicle crash is composed of three collisions that combine to produce injury. The first collision occurs when the vehicle strikes an object. The vehicle immediately undergoes a change in speed, but the occupants are still moving at the original speed until they strike the interior of the vehicle, producing the second collision. The third collision occurs when the occupants' internal organs strike each other and the internal surfaces of the body.

199. The answer is A. (Mosby/ACEP, *Truncal Trauma.*) Frontal impact motor vehicle crashes produce the largest deceleration forces. Deceleration causes the aorta to be pulled and stretched to such an extent that it may rupture at the point where ligaments are attached to it.

200. The answer is B. (Brady, *Head, Neck, and Spine Trauma.*) Patients who fall from heights greater than 15 feet are likely to land feet first, causing injury to the heels. Fractures of the calcanei are a sign that patients have fallen from a substantial height and are likely to have other serious injuries.

201. The answer is C. (Brady, *The Kinetics of Trauma.*) The pressure wave from an explosion moves through the air. Hollow, air-filled organs, such as the lungs and those of the gastrointestinal tract, are likely to be injured as the pressure wave moves through them. Solid organs and bones are less likely to be injured from the pressure wave.

202. The answer is C. (Caroline/Little Brown, *Mechanisms of Trauma.*) A medium-velocity handgun bullet is likely to create a wound channel that is twice the diameter of the bullet as it dissipates its energy through the tissues. A low-velocity projectile, such as a knife, will create tissue damage of the same diameter as the projectile. A high-velocity rifle bullet that contains massive amounts of energy may create tissue damage along a wound track 20 times the diameter of the bullet.

203. The answer is B. (Caroline/Little Brown, *Multiple Injuries: Summary of ATLS.*) Although there is some variation, the presence of a radial pulse usually indicates a systolic blood pressure of at least 80 mmHg.

204. The answer is B. (Brady, *Pathophysiology of Shock.*) Normal peripheral capillary refill should occur in less than 2 seconds. A delayed capillary refill is a sign of circulatory compromise.

205. The answer is B. (Mosby/ACEP, *Truncal Trauma.*) A collection of air under the skin, known as subcutaneous emphysema, will cause crepitus to be felt upon palpation. Decreased breath sounds and dyspnea are signs of hemothorax, electrocardiographic (ECG) changes are used to diagnose cardiac contusion, and aortic rupture is seen as profound hypotension after a deceleration injury.

206. The answer is C. (Mosby, *Airway and Ventilation.*) A two-handed technique may be required to obtain an adequate mask seal while maintaining a jaw thrust without compromising spinal immobilization. This necessitates a second person to operate the bag. A patient can be ventilated very effectively with this method. The bag-valve-mask can be used on a patient with thoracic injury, but there is an increased risk of tension pneumothorax.

207. The answer is D. (Mosby, *Trauma.*) Bleeding from a ruptured spleen may cause irritation to the diaphragm on the left side, causing a referred pain to the left shoulder. Injury to the liver typically causes right upper quadrant pain, a fracture of C_1 will cause neck pain near the base of the skull, and a hemothorax will cause chest pain and difficulty breathing.

208. The answer is C. (Mosby/ACEP, *Truncal Trauma.*) A tension pneumothorax may cause a displacement of the great veins of the chest. The resultant venous obstruction will cause distension of the neck veins. Injury to the cervical spine, hemothorax, and shock are more likely to involve an actual or relative hypovolemia, which will cause flattened neck veins.

209. The answer is A. (Brady, *Airway Management and Ventilation.*) The modified jaw thrust is the best method for initially managing the airway of a trauma patient. This method allows the airway to be maintained without significant movement of the cervical spine. The head tilt, chin lift; head tilt, neck lift; or triple airway maneuver involve tilting the head, causing significant movement of the cervical spine.

210. The answer is B. (Caroline/Little Brown, *Chest Injuries.*) A tension pneumothorax results from an expansion of air in the pleural space on the injured side. This expansion will push the structures of the mediastinum, including the trachea, toward the uninjured side.

211. The answer is D. (Mosby, *Trauma.*) Dysrhythmias caused by cardiac contusion should be treated pharmacologically in the same way as a myocardial infarction. In the case of premature ventricular contractions, lidocaine is the drug of choice. MAST trousers and rapid infusions of IV fluids should be used with caution in cases of cardiac contusion because of the chance of heart failure. Oxygen should be administered, but ventilation should be maintained normally.

212. The answer is A. (Mosby, *Trauma.*) Severe cases of flail chest, where the chest wall instability interferes with ventilation, should be managed with positive-pressure ventilation. Cricothyrotomy should only be considered in cases where an airway cannot be maintained by other means. Manual stabilization may not be effective in severe cases. Needle decompression should be used if there is a suspicion of tension pneumothorax.

213. The answer is B. (Caroline/Little Brown, *Injuries to the Head, Neck, and Spine.*) Eye opening to verbal stimulation receives 3 points for eye response. Disoriented speech receives 4 points for verbal response. Localizing pain receives 5 points for motor response. The total number of points is 12.

214. The answer is D. (Mosby, *Trauma.*) A cardiac contusion presents with chest pain similar to that of a myocardial infarction. Since cardiac muscle has been damaged, the complications of cardiac contusion are similar to those seen in myocardial infarction, such as dysrhythmias and heart failure. Pulmonary contusion presents as dyspnea and lung congestion. Aortic rupture will cause profound shock or sudden death. Muffled heart sounds, distended neck veins, and narrowed pulse pressure are seen with pericardial tamponade.

215. The answer is A. (Caroline/Little Brown, *Multiple Injuries: Summary of ATLS.*) Many critical trauma patients require immediate surgical management. In order to move the patient as rapidly as possible to the operating room, time spent on the scene should be minimized. Scene times of 10 minutes or less are optimal.

216. The answer is B. (Caroline/Little Brown, *Mechanisms of Trauma.*) Using the formula for kinetic energy, $E = mv^2$, velocity (v) is the most significant factor. Doubling the mass (m) will double the amount of energy, but doubling the velocity will increase the amount of energy four times.

217. The answer is C. (Mosby/ACEP, *Truncal Trauma.*) Internal bleeding in the abdomen will cause irritation to the peritoneum. The patient will experience abdominal distention, tenderness, and guarding to palpation. Eventually the abdominal muscles will become rigid. Injury to the superficial abdominal wall may cause some tenderness, but not guarding or rigidity. Anxiety and shock do not normally cause abdominal pain.

218. The answer is C. (Caroline/Little Brown, *Wounds and Burns.*) Patients trapped in a confined space with a fire are at high risk for airway and respiratory burns. Dyspnea, hoarseness, and facial burns are signs of airway injury. This may lead to airway obstruction due to edema. Endotracheal intubation is the appropriate immediate treatment. Intravenous fluid replacement will not help this airway problem. Burn patients should not receive anything by mouth. Sedation with diazepam should only be used if necessary to accomplish intubation.

219. The answer is B. (Mosby/ACEP, *Burn Injuries.*) Electricity tends to follow a path through the body to ground. There are often wounds where the electricity enters and exits the body. The burn injury will often extend deeply into the tissues of the body far from the wounds. There is a danger of cardiac dysrhythmia and respiratory paralysis as a result of electrical injury.

220. The answer is D. (Mosby, *Trauma.*) As a high-velocity bullet moves through the tissues of the body, it builds up a shock wave and pushes tissues ahead of it. The elastic skin on the other side of the body stretches outward until it tears in an irregularly shaped wound as the bullet bursts outward.

221. The answer is A. (Mosby, *Trauma.*) Almost all external bleeding can be controlled with direct pressure. Pressure should be applied to the wound with a dressing until bleeding stops. New dressings should be placed atop blood-soaked dressings without removing them. Once bleeding is controlled, the dressings should be held in place with a pressure dressing. Elevating the effective limb may help. A tourniquet should be reserved as a last resort if pressure and elevation fail. Vascular clamps are not used in the prehospital setting.

222. The answer is C. (Mosby, *Trauma.*) Facial injuries may cause airway obstruction due to bleeding, swelling, and displaced structures. Patients with facial injuries should be carefully monitored for airway patency. Shock is not common from isolated facial injuries. While they are serious problems, pain and disfigurement are not life threatening.

223. The answer is D. (Mosby/ACEP, *Truncal Trauma.*) The most important treatment for hypovolemic shock is bleeding control. This may be accomplished by direct pressure for external bleeding or rapid transport to the operating room for internal bleeding. Intravenous fluid replacement should be started and MAST trousers considered for profound shock. Vasopressor drugs are not useful unless intravascular volume has been replaced.

224. The answer is A. (Mosby/ACEP, *Truncal Trauma.*) The mechanism of injury, taking into account the speed, deceleration, and direction of impact, is the best clue to determining the type and severity of injuries. Much of this information may be gathered by examining the vehicles involved in the crash. The amount of debris, other injuries, and skid marks do not give as much information about the energy absorbed by the victims.

225. The answer is B. (Brady, *The Kinetics of Trauma.*) Many critical trauma patients require immediate surgical management. In order to move the patient as rapidly as possible to the operating room, time spent on the scene should be minimized. Scene times of 10 minutes or less are optimal.

226. **The answer is A.** (Brady, *The Kinetics of Trauma.*) The decision to move immediately or attempt on-scene care is critical. The most common preventable causes of mortality in trauma patients are asphyxia and hemorrhage. All on-scene care should be aimed at securing an airway, maintaining an airway, and controlling bleeding.

227. **The answer is D.** (Brady, *The Kinetics of Trauma.*) The release of energy is what causes injury in trauma. Using the formula $E = mv^2$, a 2000-lb car moving at 30 mph will have 900,000 units of energy. If we double the speed to 60 mph, the energy will rise to 3,600,000 units.

228. **The answer is B.** (Mosby/ACEP, *Truncal Trauma.*) In blunt trauma, the internal organs are displaced and may strike each other or the internal wall of the body. The solid organs that have more mass are particularly vulnerable to injury as a result of this motion.

229. **The answer is B.** (Mosby, *Trauma.*) Rear-impact collisions may cause the head to be hyperextended backward over the rear seat, causing injury to the cervical spine and muscles of the neck. This is especially true if the head rests are not properly adjusted.

230. **The answer is A.** (Brady, *The Kinetics of Trauma.*) Hollow-point and soft-tipped bullets are designed to spread out upon impact, increasing the frontal profile of the bullet. This causes the wound channel to be larger and more energy to be transferred to the victim.

231. **The answer is A.** (Brady, *The Kinetics of Trauma.*) As a firearm is discharged, hot gases and unburned and partially burned gunpowder are also ejected from the barrel. A victim at close range will be sprayed with gas and gunpowder, causing burns and tattooing around the wound. This is seen regardless of the type of weapon or ammunition.

232. **The answer is A.** (Mosby/ACEP, *HEENT Trauma.*) No attempt should be made to stop the flow of cerebrospinal fluid from nose or ears. Packing of the ears or nose may cause a buildup of intracranial pressure.

233. **The answer is C.** (Brady, *Head, Neck, and Spine Injury.*) The term *contrecoup* is used to describe an injury that occurs when the brain strikes the inside of the skull on the side opposite to the original impact. An epidural hematoma is a collection of blood between the skull and dura mater. A subdural hematoma is a collection of blood between the dura mater and the brain. A concussion is a transient loss of consciousness due to a blow to the head.

234. **The answer is A.** (Mosby/ACEP, *HEENT Trauma.*) A hyphema is a collection of blood that may be seen in front of a patient's pupil and iris due to a direct trauma to the eye.

235. **The answer is D.** (Mosby, *Trauma.*) Manual stabilization must be maintained until the patient has been immobilized to a spine board. A cervical collar alone does not provide adequate immobilization. Proper stabilization should reduce pain and must be maintained.

236. **The answer is A.** (Caroline/Little Brown, *Injuries to the Head, Neck, and Spine.*) Intubation attempts may cause gagging and hypoxia, which may lead to dysrhythmias and increased intracranial pressure. Adequate preoxygenation, intravenous lidocaine, and sedation as necessary will help to avoid these complications.

237. **The answer is A.** (Mosby/ACEP, *HEENT Trauma.*) Mild hyperventilation will lower $Paco_2$, causing cerebral vasoconstriction, thereby decreasing cerebral blood flow. This may be useful in preventing increased intracranial pressure. However, hyperventilation should be reserved for those patients showing signs of increased intracranial pressure. Reducing cerebral blood flow may be harmful for patients in the early stages of head injury.

238. **The answer is A.** (Mosby, *Trauma.*) Arterial bleeding from the neck should be controlled with direct pressure. Care must be taken so as not to create an airway obstruction. Tourniquets and tight bandages would cause an airway obstruction and are inappropriate in the management of neck wounds. Venous bleeding from the neck should be managed with an occlusive dressing to prevent air embolism.

239. **The answer is A.** (Caroline/Little Brown, *Injuries to the Head, Neck, and Spine.*) Head injuries may affect the body's temperature-regulating mechanism. This may result in hypothermia or hyperthermia. Spinal injuries that may accompany serious head injuries may also cause hypothermia due to vasodilation from decreased sympathetic tone.

240. **The answer is B.** (Caroline/Little Brown, *Injuries to the Head, Neck, and Spine.*) A protective cup should be secured over an object impaled in the eye to prevent movement and further injury. Tight dressings should be avoided because they may force the object deeper or collapse the globe. Impaled objects in the eye should never be removed. A loose dressing may not prevent movement of the object.

241. **The answer is B.** (Caroline/Little Brown, *Chest Injuries.*) Under normal circumstances, the pressure between the visceral and parietal pleura is lower than atmospheric pressure. This causes the lungs to expand and fill the space completely. In certain types of illness or injury, air or fluid may collect in the pleural space. The diaphragm lies beneath the lungs.

242. **The answer is A.** (Caroline/Little Brown, *Injuries to the Abdomen and GU Tract.*) Flank pain and blood in the urine are signs of injury to the kidney. Pain in the right upper quadrant is a sign of injury to the liver. Pain in the left upper quadrant referred to the left shoulder is a sign of injury to the spleen. Injury to the heart will cause pain in the anterior part of the chest.

243. The answer is C. (Caroline/Little Brown, *Injuries to the Abdomen and GU Tract.*) During respiration, the diaphragm rises and falls, exposing the thoracic and abdominal organs to injury from a penetration at the level of the lower rib margin. A wound may also extend through the diaphragm and cause injuries to the thoracic and abdominal organs simultaneously. It is unlikely that a stab wound to the anterior surface of the body would cause injury to the spine.

244. The answer is C. (Caroline/Little Brown, *Chest Injuries.*) Immobilizing rib fractures will limit the expansion of the chest. This may help relieve some pain and stabilize a flail chest. However, the decreased expansion of the lungs will impair the exchange of air and may lead to the collapse of alveoli. This will make the patient more susceptible to a pneumonia.

245. The answer is A. (Brady, *Body Cavity Trauma.*) A flail segment of the chest will exhibit a motion known as paradoxical respiration. The flail segment will move in the direction opposite to that of the rest of the ribcage. During inspiration, the ribcage will be seen to expand outward, and the flail segment will collapse inward. During expiration, the rib cage will move inward, and the flail segment will balloon outward.

246. The answer is C. (Brady, *Body Cavity Trauma.*) Frothy blood bubbling from a chest wound is often referred to as a "sucking" chest wound. There is a direct opening for air to pass into the chest. This is an open pneumothorax. Paradoxical movement of a section of the chest wall is seen with flail chest. Diminished breath sounds at the bases of the lung fields and signs of shock are seen with hemothorax. A patient with a tension pneumothorax will have diminished breath sounds and tracheal deviation.

247. The answer is A. (Caroline/Little Brown, *Chest Injuries.*) Severe difficulty breathing and shock are signs of tension pneumothorax. The diagnosis can be confirmed by examining for diminished breath sounds and tracheal deviation. A ruptured aorta would present with profound hemorrhagic shock. Intraabdominal bleeding would cause tenderness and rigidity of the abdomen. Traumatic asphyxia results from severe compression of the chest and is diagnosed by the presence of severe venous congestion in the face.

248. The answer is B. (Caroline/Little Brown, *Chest Injuries.*) If blood collects in the pericardial sac surrounding the heart, it may compress the heart and prevent it from filling normally. This condition is known as pericardial tamponade. A myocardial infarction is the death of heart muscle due to a lack of oxygen. A cardiomyopathy is a nonspecific disease of heart muscle. Congestive heart failure results from a weakened heart muscle.

249. The answer is D. (Brady, *Body Cavity Trauma.*) Jugular vein distention, a narrowed pulse pressure, and a rapid thready pulse are signs of pericardial tamponade. Muffled heart sounds is another sign that is commonly seen with pericardial tamponade. Tracheal deviation is seen with tension pnuemothorax because the lungs are displaced toward the uninjured side.

250. The answer is B. (Caroline/Little Brown, *Chest Injuries.*) If there is no sign of spinal injury that would require immobilization, a patient with a chest injury is best transported lying on the injured side. In this case, gravity will help to prevent the displacement of the heart and great vessels if a tension pneumothorax should develop. The Trendelenburg position would be very uncomfortable, and pressure from the abdominal organs may interfere with the movement of the diaphragm.

251. The answer is A. (Mosby, *Trauma.*) Over the top of the third rib in the second intercostal space is the correct location for a pleural decompression. This location is most likely to release any trapped air and avoid any damage to internal organs or major blood vessels.

252. The answer is C. (Mosby, *Trauma.*) Air is being trapped in the chest, and the patient is developing a tension pneumothorax. Unsealing the wound will allow the air to be released. Leaving an open side to occlusive dressings may allow air to escape and prevent this problem. Intubation and hyperventilation will introduce large amounts of air into the chest and are likely to make this problem worse. Transporting a patient on the injured side may relieve some of the organ displacement that results from a tension pneumothorax. High-concentration oxygen would be helpful, but it is more important to relieve the tension pneumothorax.

253. The answer is D. (Mosby/ACEP, *Truncal Trauma.*) Blunt force trauma to the anterior chest may cause a contusion to the cardiac muscle. The injured myocardium is prone to dysrhythmias and complications similar to a myocardial infarction. Patients with suspected myocardial contusion should have continuous ECG monitoring. Dysrhythmias should be managed with the same medications as a myocardial infarction.

254. The answer is A. (Brady, *Body Cavity Trauma.*) Removal of an impaled object may cause additional damage. Impaled objects should be stabilized as they are found with bulky dressings. If there is obvious air leakage, an occlusive dressing should be packed around the object. The only exception is for objects impaled in the cheek that may interfere with the airway. These may be carefully removed. A needle decompression should only be performed if there are signs of tension pneumothorax.

255. The answer is D. (Caroline/Little Brown, *Injuries to the Abdomen and GU Tract.*) Organs protruding from the abdomen should be covered with a sterile dressing moistened with sterile normal saline solution. The organs should not be allowed to dry in the air or be covered with a dry dressing that would wick moisture away from the organs. No attempt should be made to replace protruding organs into the body.

256. The answer is B. (Mosby, *Trauma.*) If a joint is moved beyond its normal range of motion, an injury to ligaments and other connective tissues that surround the joint may occur. This is known as a sprain. A strain is an injury that occurs to a muscle that has been overstressed. A dislocation occurs when the bones of joint are forced out of their normal position. A contusion is a soft-tissue injury that results from blunt force trauma.

257. **The answer is C.** (Brady, *Musculoskeletal Injuries.*) Dislocations should be immobilized to prevent further injury. In order to properly immobilize a joint, it is necessary to include the bone above and the bone below the joint in the immobilizaton.

258. **The answer is D.** (Mosby/ACEP, *Orthopedic Injuries.*) A fracture of the femur may cause life-threatening hemorrhage. The rich blood supply of the surrounding tissues and the proximity of the femoral artery make fractures of the femur more likely to cause severe bleeding. In addition, the patient may lose large amounts of blood into the thigh without its being obvious.

259. **The answer is A.** (Brady, *Musculoskeletal Injuries.*) A pelvic fracture may involve injury to major blood vessels, and instability of the pelvis creates a large area for blood to collect. Injury to the bladder is often seen with pelvic fracture, but this is not life threatening. Severe deformities and paralysis are not common with a fractured pelvis.

260. **The answer is C.** (Mosby, *Trauma.*) A loss of pulses after applying a splint is most likely caused by excessive pressure from the splint on the extremity. The simplest way to manage this is to loosen the splint and recheck the pulse. If this fails, it may be necessary to reposition the splint. If a pulse is still not detected, the patient should be transported to the hospital.

261. **The answer is D.** (Brady, *Musculoskeletal Injuries.*) If resistance is met while attempting to realign a fracture, no further attempt should be made to straighten the limb. Applying more force or further manipulation is likely to cause further injury.

262. **The answer is B.** (Brady, *Musculoskeletal Injuries.*) Dislocated joints should be splinted in the position in which they are found. An exception to this is when there is circulatory or neurological compromise. In this case, one attempt at gentle manipulation of the limb should be made in an effort to restore circulation and neurological function.

263. **The answer is A.** (Brady, *Musculoskeletal Injuries.*) A traction splint is the most effective method of immobilizing a fractured femur. The traction splint will prevent the bone ends from moving due to the spasm of the large muscles of the thigh. This will prevent additional injury to the structures surrounding the femur. The PASG will not be able to hold the limb in alignment against the spasm of the muscles. An air splint will not extend to include the hip joint. Rigid board splints may be used, but they will not be able to hold the bone in alignment as well as the traction splint.

264. **The answer is D.** (Caroline/Little Brown, *Fractures, Dislocations, and Sprains.*) A pillow may be used to splint the irregular bones of the ankle. The pillow should be wrapped around the ankle and secured with cravats or a bandage. A pillow will not provide adequate rigidity to splint long bones such as the femur and humerus.

265. **The answer is A.** (Mosby, *Soft-Tissue and Burns.*) When an injury to blood vessels causes a collection of blood beneath the skin, this is known as a hematoma. A contusion is an injury to soft tissue caused by blunt force trauma. A laceration is a jagged open wound caused by a tearing force applied to the skin. An abrasion is an open wound caused by friction applied to the skin.

266. **The answer is B.** (Mosby, *Soft-Tissue Injuries and Wounds.*) A puncture wound allows bacteria to be introduced deep under the skin. The beginning of the healing process will exclude oxygen from the inside of the wound. This may create a favorable environment for anaerobic bacteria to grow.

267. **The answer is B.** (Mosby, *Soft Tissue Injuries and Burns.*) An avulsion is a wound where soft tissue has been torn away. An avulsion may be complete when the tissue is completely separated from the body or partial when it remains connected by a flap. A contusion is a soft-tissue injury from blunt force. An abrasion is an open wound caused by friction. An amputation occurs when a portion of the body containing a bone has been torn away.

268. **The answer is A.** (Mosby, *Soft Tissue Injuries and Burns.*) Tearing forces applied to the skin will create an open wound with jagged edges, known as a laceration. An incision is a wound with smooth edges created by a sharp object. An abrasion is an open wound caused by friction against the skin. A puncture is created when a pointed object protrudes deep under the skin.

269. **The answer is D.** (Caroline/Little Brown, *Wounds and Burns.*) Carbon monoxide is a common product of incomplete combustion. The carbon monoxide levels in an enclosed space with a fire will rise rapidly. Most fatalities in fires result from carbon monoxide poisoning. Cyanide poisoning may result from the burning of certain plastics. Thermal burns and systemic heat stroke will not occur unless the victim is exposed for a longer period of time.

270. **The answer is A.** (Caroline/Little Brown, *Wounds and Burns.*) Third-degree burns extend through the full thickness of the dermis. As a result, the nerve endings that would normally perceive pain are destroyed. First-degree burns and some second-degree burns do not involve blisters. Third-degree burns may appear brown, red, black, or white, depending on the source of the burn. The surface of a third-degree burn appears dry.

271. **The answer is D.** (Caroline/Little Brown, *Wounds and Burns.*) Burns around the mouth and nose are a sign of burns to the airway and inhalation of hot gases that will damage the lungs. Airway and respiratory compromise are among the most serious complications of burn injury.

272. **The answer is C.** (Caroline/Little Brown, *Wounds and Burns.*) Pressure on the brachial artery, located in the medial upper arm, may help to control bleeding from the area of the wrist. The femoral pressure point in the groin may be used for bleeding in the upper leg. The temporal pressure point on the skull may be used for bleeding from the scalp. The popliteal pressure point behind the knee may be used to help control bleeding in the lower leg.

273. **The answer is D.** (Caroline/Little Brown, *Wounds and Burns.*) Ringer's lactate is the preferred solution for fluid replacement for burn injury. Ringer's lactate supplies more of the electrolytes that are lost from the burn injury.

274. **The answer is C.** (Mosby, *Soft Tissue Injuries and Burns.*) Chemical burn injuries should be irrigated with copious amounts of water for at least 20 minutes to ensure that all chemical has been removed from the skin. Some exceptions are phenol, which should be irrigated with alcohol, and dry chemicals, which should be brushed off prior to irrigation with water. Neutralizing agents should not be applied to a patient because they will cause a chemical reaction that will release heat and gasses.

275. **The answer is C.** (Brady, *Soft Tissue Trauma and Burns.*) Phenol (carbolic acid) is a caustic substance that is not soluble in water. Irrigation with water will not be effective. Phenol is soluble in alcohol. Irrigation with alcohol will help to remove phenol from the skin.

276. **The answer is B.** (Brady, *Soft Tissue Trauma and Burns.*) Dry caustic chemicals should be managed by brushing as much of the chemical away as possible prior to irrigating with water. Some dry chemicals are activated by water, and irrigating first may cause more damage. Neutralizing agents such as baking soda may cause a chemical reaction that will release heat and gases. Alcohol should only be used to irrigate contamination with phenol.

277. **The answer is D.** (Caroline/Little Brown, *Injuries to the Head, Neck, and Spine.*) Patients with spinal injuries tend to have normal or slow pulses. Spinal injuries are often accompanied by dysfunction of the sympathetic nervous system. This will prevent the patient's pulse rate from rising. A spider crack in the windshield and contusion on the patient's forehead are signs of axial loading that may lead to spinal injury. Numbness and tingling of the extremities are signs that there may be injury to the spinal cord.

278. **The answer is A.** (Brady, *Comprehensive Patient Assessment.*) A patient with a lumbar spine injury is not likely to deteriorate or require immediate surgery. Spinal injury patients benefit from careful, deliberate transportation. Patients with signs of shock may have internal bleeding that will benefit from immediate surgery. An unstable pelvic fracture may cause severe internal bleeding. A deteriorating mental status may indicate a severe injury to the central nervous system.

279. **The answer is B.** (Caroline/Little Brown, *Fractures, Dislocations, and Sprains.*) Most bleeding from an amputation can be controlled with direct pressure, elevation, and pressure points. A tourniquet should be used as a last resort. A tourniquet may cause more of the limb to be lost.

280. **The answer is D.** (Mosby, *Trauma.*) A spinal injury may affect the nerves that suppress an erection. In these cases, a patient would have a persistent erection, known as priapism.

281. The answer is B. (Mosby, *Trauma.*) You should fill any voids with a noncompressible padding, such as folding sheets, in order to better stabilize the patient. The patient will not be any more likely to conform to the short board. You should never attempt to force a patient down to the board. By doing this, you would be likely to create more injuries.

282. The answer is C. (Mosby, *Trauma.*) Sandbags are cheap and easy to use, and will hold the patient's head securely as long as the backboard remains level. If the backboard is tilted to the side, the weight of the sandbags may push the patient's head to the side, compromising spinal immobilization.

283. The answer is B. (Brady, *Head, Neck, and Spine Injury.*) Performing the jaw thrust while maintaining in-line stabilization is the safest and most effective initial method of managing the airway of a trauma patient. Endotracheal intubation should be utilized after simpler methods have been employed. The head tilt, chin lift will cause excessive movement of the cervical spine. The esophageal obturator airway should not be used in patients less that 16 years of age.

284. The answer is A. (Brady, *Head, Neck, and Spine Injury.*) You should record the patient's motor and sensory functions prior to extrication from a crashed automobile. This will serve as documentation of the patient's condition prior to the manipulation necessary to remove a patient from an automobile.

285. The answer is B. (Caroline/Little Brown, *Injuries to the Abdomen and GU Tract.*) The tenderness of the abdomen indicates the possibility of an intraabdominal bleed. Deceleration injuries seen in frontal collisions are likely to cause trauma to the solid organs of the abdomen with internal bleeding. The chest examination did not reveal any signs of pulmonary compromise. Tension pneumothorax and pericardial tamponade cause distended neck veins.

286. The answer is B. (Mosby/ACEP, *Orthopedic Injuries.*) Pain in the right thigh with shortening and external rotation of the limb are classic signs of femur fracture. Femur fractures are best managed with a traction splint that will move the bone ends back into alignment. A pillow splint would not provide enough support for a fractured femur. A sling and swathe is used for an upper arm. If a traction splint is not available, the fractured leg may be secured to the uninjured leg.

287. The answer is A. (Mosby, *Trauma.*) The nasal bones are small and unprotected. Blows to the frontal face area tend to strike the nose first.

288. The answer is B. (Brady, *Head, Neck, and Spine Injury.*) The patient has signs of upper airway obstruction. A fracture of the cartilages making up the larynx will cause airway obstruction due to swelling and displacement of structures. A zygoma fracture would be seen as a deformity to the face. An aortic disruption would cause sudden and severe shock. A simple pneumothorax would cause shortness of breath and diminished breath sounds.

289. **The answer is C.** (Brady, *Head, Neck, and Spine Injury.*) The maxilla is located in the lower third of the face and the upper jaw. The ethmoid is located in the skull, between the eyes. The mandible is the lower jaw. The zygoma is the upper and outer cheek.

290. **The answer is C.** (Mosby, *Trauma.*) Increased intracranial pressure may affect the respiratory control centers of the brain stem, causing changes in breathing patterns. Rising intracranial pressure will cause a decrease in mental alertness, hypertension, and bradycardia. If a head injury patient appears with hypotension and tachycardia, it is usually the result of bleeding somewhere else in the body.

291. **The answer is C.** (Mosby, *Trauma.*) Bilateral periorbital ecchymosis (two black eyes) are sometimes referred to as raccoon's eyes. This is a sign of basal skull fracture. Battle's sign is ecchymosis behind the ear and is also a sign of basal skull fracture. Cullen's sign is ecchymosis around the navel, associated with abdominal bleeding. McBurney's sign is abdominal pain and tenderness in the right lower quadrant.

292. **The answer is D.** (Caroline/Little Brown, *Injuries to the Head, Neck, and Spine.*) A score of 15 on the Glasgow coma scale is normal. A score of 3 would indicate complete unresponsiveness. Scores below 8 are recognized to represent coma.

293. **The answer is C.** (Brady, *Musculoskeletal Injuries.*) An injured hand should be immobilized in the position of function, with the fingers slightly flexed around a roll of gauze in the hand. This will keep stress off the structures of the injured hand.

294. **The answer is C.** (Brady, *The Kinetics of Trauma.*) When a patient strikes his or her head against the windshield of an automobile, significant force is applied down the length of the spine. This is known as axial loading. As a result, there may be a significant chance of spinal injury.

295. **The answer is A.** (Mosby, *Trauma.*) Fractures of the temporal and parietal skull may cause a disruption of the middle cerebral artery. This will cause arterial bleeding between the skull and the dura mater. An intraventricular hemorrhage is a bleed that occurs deep within the brain. A subdural hematoma is a collection of venous blood between the dura mater and the brain. A subarachnoid hemorrhage is bleeding at the base of the brain that most commonly occurs as a result of the spontaneous rupture of an aneurysm at the base of the brain.

296. **The answer is A.** (Brady, *Pathophysiology of Shock.*) Pale skin, tachycardia, and hypotension are classical signs of hypovolemic shock. Flushed skin is often seen with certain types of shock, such as anaphylactic shock.

297. **The answer is B.** (Mosby, *Obstetrical and Neonatal Emergencies.*) In cases of near-term pregnancy, the gravid uterus will press on the inferior vena cava while the patient lies supine. This may reduce the venous return to the heart and aggravate hypovolemia caused by trauma. Whenever possible, trauma patients who are pregnant near term should be transported in the left lateral recumbent position. In addition to improving the venous return, this position allows for better circulation to the fetus.

298. **The answer is D.** (Brady, *Shock Trauma Resuscitation.*) If at all possible, trauma patients should receive two large-bore IVs. However, time should not be wasted at the scene starting IVs. If the patient can be rapidly moved to the ambulance, the IVs are best started while en route to the hospital. Intravenous fluids should be run only at a rate sufficient to prevent hypotension.

SECTION V:
PATIENT PRESENTATIONS: MEDICAL

The following topics are covered in Section V:

- Medical Pulmonary
- Medical Cardiology
- Medical Neurology
- Endocrine Emergencies
- Anaphylaxis
- Gastroenterology
- Renal and Urology
- Toxicology
- Hematology
- Environmental Emergencies
- Infectious and Communicable Diseases
- Behavioral and Psychiatric Disorders
- Gynecologic Emergencies
- Obstetrics

MEDICAL
PULMONARY

Directions: Each item below contains four suggested responses. Select the **one best** response to each item.

299. All of the following are signs of impending respiratory failure EXCEPT

(A) nasal flaring and tracheal tugging
(B) cyanosis
(C) respiratory rate greater than 18 breaths per minute or less than 12 breaths per minute in an adult
(D) accessory muscle use

300. You begin to evaluate a 34-year-old female with a long history of asthma who is complaining of increasing difficulty breathing for the past 5 days. The patient notes that she caught a cold about a week ago and has been getting worse ever since. She is having difficulty speaking in complete sentences but does note that she has taken her inhaler medications several times a day, without improvement. Which of the following findings on auscultation is the most critical in this patient?

(A) mild expiratory wheezing
(B) severe inspiratory and expiratory wheezing
(C) silent chest
(D) diffuse bilateral rhonchi

301. You are dispatched to a 28-year-old male who is complaining of difficulty breathing. He has a 10-year history of asthma and has been under the care of a primary-care physician. He has been taking a number of medications daily yet notes that the onset of the hay fever season has played a significant part in worsening his breathing. As you assess the patient, you note that his vital signs are a blood pressure of 140/78, a pulse of 102 per minute, and a respiratory rate of 34 breaths per minute. With medical control approval, all of the following are acute emergency care treatments available to you for treating this asthmatic patient EXCEPT

(A) nasal oxygen at 2 to 3 liters/minute
(B) beta-agonist oral inhalers
(C) subcutaneous epinephrine
(D) intravenous (IV) corticosteroids

302. The pathology of the airways in asthma includes all of the following EXCEPT

(A) edema
(B) secretions
(C) inflammation
(D) blood

303. All of the following are medications that physicians commonly prescribe for the outpatient treatment of asthmatic patients EXCEPT

(A) the oral beta-agonist inhalers labeled albuterol, metaproterenol, isoetharine, and terbutaline
(B) oral prednisone, oral prednisolone, and various steroid inhalers
(C) oral aminophylline preparations
(D) oral anti-inflammatory agents

304. Which of the following items is specifically helpful for evaluating the asthmatic patient at home, in the pre-hospital setting by the Paramedic, in the emergency department, and in the hospital units?

(A) pulse oximeter
(B) arterial blood gas determinations
(C) peak expiratory flow rate meter
(D) electrocardiogram (ECG)

305. All of the following are conditions associated with chronic obstructive pulmonary disease (COPD) EXCEPT

(A) emphysema
(B) cor pulmonale
(C) chronic bronchitis
(D) pneumonia

306. You are dispatched to a 70-year-old male, at home, with difficulty breathing. As you arrive at the patient's home, the patient's wife tells you that the patient has chronic lung disease due to smoking 3 packs of cigarettes a day for 40 years. The patient had a cold 2 weeks ago and has continued to have more difficulty breathing over this period of time. The patient has had difficulty even walking to the bathroom and around the apartment. Last month he was able to walk a couple of blocks outside, with feeling a little short of breath but nothing as dramatic as this. Upon examining the patient, you note that he is sitting upright in a chair and leaning forward, with his arms holding the bottom of the chair. The patient's lips and nail beds are cyanotic, and he is breathing at 34 breaths per minute, with a blood pressure of 112/68, a regular pulse of 92, supraclavicular retractions, and pursed-lip breathing. All of the following are parts of the acute management of this patient EXCEPT

(A) nasal oxygen at 2 to 3 liters/minute
(B) subcutaneous (SC) epinephrine 0.3 mg
(C) IV line to keep a vein open
(D) albuterol or metaproterenol oral inhaler

307. You are stationed at a state fair when a frightened teenager runs over to you saying that her friend is complaining of chest pain and shortness of breath. As you walk over to the 17-year-old male, sitting on a bench, he states that he was simply walking around the fair with his girlfriend when he developed the acute onset of dyspnea, pleuritic chest pain, and tachypnea. Your assessment reveals that the patient has no breath sounds in the symptomatic area of his chest. The treatment of choice for this patient includes which of the following?

(A) needle decompression of the chest
(B) beta-agonist oral inhaler
(C) SC epinephrine 0.3 mg
(D) 100 percent oxygen by non-rebreather mask

308. An acute pulmonary disease that produces noncardiogenic pulmonary edema and severe hypoxemia, and is brought about by increased capillary permeability in the pulmonary arterial system is known as

(A) asthma
(B) adult respiratory distress syndrome
(C) acute pulmonary embolism
(D) hyperventilation syndrome

309. You are dispatched to the home of a 22-year-old male who is complaining of severe dizziness and is breathing rapidly. As you arrive at the patient's home, you are told that there was a loud, angry argument between the patient's parents and that the patient became very upset and began to breathe rapidly. He is dizzy, is unable to catch his breath, and feels numbness and tingling in his hands and feet. Upon examination, you note that the patient's lungs are bilaterally clear, without rales, rhonchi, or wheezes, and with very good aeration bilaterally. The correct emergent treatment of this patient includes which of the following?

(A) allowing the patient to simply rebreathe in a paper bag
(B) administering oxygen and trying to reassure the patient
(C) administering a beta-agonist oral inhaler
(D) administering IV furosemide

310. All of the following are medications that are prescribed by physicians for patients suffering from difficulty breathing due to various diseases EXCEPT

(A) aminophylline tablets, oral beta-agonist inhalers, oral steroid inhalers, and oral steroid tablets
(B) digoxin tablets; nitroglycerin tablets, spray, paste, or patches; furosemide tablets; Isordil tablets; Captopril tablets; Enalopril tablets; and aspirin
(C) Coumadin tablets and heparin injections
(D) Pepcid, Zantac, Axid, Prilosec, Prevacid, and Tagamet

311. While driving to pick up lunch, you are dispatched to a "difficulty breathing" patient in a fourth-story walk-up apartment. As you enter, you are met by the patient's husband, who states that his 83-year-old wife developed a touch of the flu about 7 days ago, never got over the cough, and developed a fever, chills, sweating, and weakness 2 days ago. This morning, when she became very short of breath, he became very worried and called for the ambulance. Your assessment of the patient reveals an elderly, diaphoretic, very weak female who is breathing 34 times per minute, is hot to the touch, has a blood pressure of 102/76, has a pulse of 130 per minute, appears to be truly dyspneic, and has a very thick, moist cough. The patient's lungs reveal dry, crisp rales in the bases of both lung fields. As you consider the possibility of pneumonia, all of the following are parts of the pre-hospital emergency care administered to this patient EXCEPT

(A) IV antibiotics
(B) opening and maintaining the airway
(C) 100 percent oxygen with a non-rebreather mask
(D) IV fluids and ECG monitoring

312. All of the following are types of pneumonia EXCEPT

(A) tuberculosis
(B) aspiration
(C) mycoplasma
(D) foreign legion

MEDICAL PULMONARY

ANSWERS

299. **The answer is C.** (Brady, *Respiratory Emergencies*; Moby/ACEP, *Dyspnea*.) (A), (B), (D), pursed lips, inability to speak, altered mental status, a pulse rate above 130 per minute or below 60 per minute in an adult, and a respiratory rate above 30 breaths per minute or below 8 breaths per minute in an adult are all signs of impending respiratory failure. (C) is incorrect.

300. **The answer is C.** (Mosby/ACEP, *Dyspnea*.) (C) is correct because markedly decreased air movement, a silent chest, is an ominous sign of respiratory failure, and the Paramedics must be prepared to support the patient's ventilation. (A) is incorrect because mild expiratory wheezing is a common finding in the mild to moderately symptomatic asthmatic patient. (B) is incorrect because loud inspiratory and expiratory wheezing is a sign of mild to moderate asthma with good air exchange. (D) is incorrect because rhonchi are usually a sign of mucous in the airways, as is present in bronchitis or pneumonia.

301. **The answer is A.** (Brady, *Respiratory Emergencies*.) (B), (C), (D), high concentration (100 percent) oxygen, and IV aminophylline are all emergency care treatments available to you. (A) is not appropriate because asthmatics complaining of difficulty breathing should be treated with high-concentration, 100 percent oxygen by nonrebreather mask.

302. **The answer is D.** (Mosby/ACEP, *Dyspnea*.) (D) is correct because blood is not part of the pathology of asthma. (A), (B), and (C) are all part of the pathology of the asthmatics' airways.

303. **The answer is D.** (Brady, *Respiratory Emergencies*.) (A), (B), and (C) are all common medications prescribed for long-term management of the asthmatic patient. (D) is the exception because there is no role for oral anti-inflammatory agents in the treatment of asthma. Some asthmatic patients with a known allergy to aspirin may actually be allergic to oral anti-inflammatory agents, and they may worsen the patient's asthma.

304. The answer is C. (Brady, *Respiratory Emergencies.*) (C) is correct because the peak expiratory flow rate (PEFR) measures the air-flow rate during maximal exhalation and is used to repetitively measure the severity of the asthmatic attack. It is also used to measure the response to treatment. (A), (B), and (C) are all important adjuncts that help to evaluate and monitor all emergently ill patients. However, the PEFR is specifically the most helpful for the acutely ill asthmatic patient.

305. The answer is D. (Brady, *Respiratory Emergencies.*) (A) and (C) are two chronic pulmonary conditions, which may, over a long period of time, cause pulmonary hypertension. Pulmonary hypertension may lead to the development of right heart failure, known as cor pulmonale (B). (D) is the exception because all patients, with or without COPD, are susceptible to the development of pneumonia, which is an infectious disease.

306. The answer is B. (Brady, *Respiratory Emergencies.*) (A), (C), and (D) are all part of the emergency treatment of the patient with decompensated COPD. (B) is not appropriate because SC epinephrine is given for the treatment of asthma, not COPD.

307. The answer is D. (Caroline/Little Brown, *Chest Injuries.*) (D) is correct because this patient's presentation is consistent with a spontaneous pneumothorax, and 100 percent oxygen, frequent checking of vital signs, and watching for the development of a tension pneumothorax are important treatment options. (A) is incorrect because this is the treatment of a confirmed tension pneumothorax, not a simple pneumothorax. (B) and (C) have no place in the treatment of a simple pneumothorax.

308. The answer is B. (Mosby, *Respiratory Disorders.*) (B) is correct and is caused as a complication of various disorders, such as trauma, infections, drug overdose, toxic gas inhalation, aspiration of gastric contents, hematologic disorders, and certain toxic metabolic disorders. Treatment involves the aggressive administration of oxygen using endotracheal intubation with the administration of positive end-expiratory pressure (PEEP), which helps to keep alveoli open by pushing fluid out of the alveoli back into the interstitium or capillaries. (A), (C), and (D) are incorrect.

309. The answer is B. (Caroline/Little Brown, *Respiratory Emergencies.*) (B) is correct because this patient demonstrates the hyperventilation syndrome. However, hyperventilation may be a part of the presentation of a number of emergent conditions, such as an acute myocardial infarction, acute pulmonary embolism, and diabetic ketoacidosis. As a result, the patient needs to be given supplemental oxygen. Allowing the patient to rebreathe in a paper bag (A), will permit the patient to raise his CO_2 levels by rebreathing his own CO_2 but may actually worsen the patient's condition by lowering his blood oxygen level. As the patient rebreathes his own exhaled air, the oxygen content of the paper bag continues to drop to very low levels. (C) and (D) have no place in the treatment of the hyperventilation syndrome.

310. The answer is D. (Mosby/ACEP, *Dyspnea.*) The medications in (A) are used for myriad pulmonary diseases, which often produce difficulty breathing, especially asthma and COPD. The medications in (B) are used to treat patients with congestive heart failure. Those in (C) are used to treat patients who have suffered pulmonary emboli and require anticoagulation. (D) includes medications primarily used to treat various gastrointestinal problems, such as peptic ulcer disease and gastroesophageal reflux disorder.

311. The answer is A. (Mosby, *Respiratory Disorders.*) (A) is correct because the administration of IV antibiotics is truly a hospital-based, nonemergent treatment. (B), (C), (D), and transportation to the emergency department are all parts of the emergent care of the patient with pneumonia.

312. The answer is D. (Mosby, *Respiratory Disorders.*) (A), (B), (C), viral, bacterial, and legionnaires' disease are all types of pneumonia. (D) is incorrect; the foreign legion is an organization, while legionnaires' disease is a type of pneumonia.

MEDICAL
CARDIOLOGY

Directions: Each item below contains four suggested responses. Select the **one best** response to each item.

313. All of the following are correct statements concerning cardiovascular disease statistics in the United States EXCEPT

(A) Cardiovascular disease is responsible for around 1 million deaths each year.

(B) About 10 percent of these deaths are due to myocardial infarctions.

(C) Diseases of the heart are primarily due to obstruction of the coronary arteries.

(D) Early cardiopulmonary resuscitation (CPR) and early advanced life support, particularly early defibrillation, have proven effective in preventing many of these deaths.

314. All of the following are known to be major risk factors predisposing to coronary artery disease EXCEPT

(A) family history of smoking

(B) cigarette smoking

(C) hypertension

(D) hypercholesterolemia

315. All of the following are correct statements about the anatomy of the heart EXCEPT

(A) The heart is located above the diaphragm, posterior to and slightly to the right of the sternum.

(B) The heart is surrounded by the pericardium and is made up of the outer-layer epicardium, the middle-layer myocardium, and the inner-layer endocardium.

(C) The four chambers of the heart consist of the right atria, right ventricle, left atria, and left ventricle.

(D) The four valves in the heart are the tricuspid (between the right atrium and right ventricle) and the pulmonary (between the right ventricle and the pulmonary artery) on the right side of the heart and the mitral (between the left atrium and the left ventricle) and aortic (between the left ventricle and the aorta) on the left side of the heart.

316. Which of the following is the correct sequence of flow of blood leaving the left ventricle?

(A) arteries, aorta, arterioles, vena cavae, venules, veins, right atrium

(B) right atrium, aorta, arteries, arterioles, venules, vena cavae, veins

(C) aorta, arteries, arterioles, venules, veins, vena cavae, right atrium

(D) arteries, aorta, arterioles, veins, vena cavae, right atrium, venules

317. Cardiac output is defined as the amount of blood that is pumped out of either ventricle in liters per minute. Which of the following is the correct formula for determining a patient's cardiac output?

(A) Blood pressure = cardiac output × peripheral resistance

(B) $E = mc^2$

(C) Cardiac output (milliliters per minute) = stroke volume (milliliters) × heart rate (beats per minute)

(D) Cardiac output = blood pressure × heart rate

318. In the normal heart, certain areas of the myocardium receive coronary artery blood supply from particular branches of the coronary arteries. All of the following are correct examples EXCEPT

(A) The left anterior descending (LAD) artery supplies blood to the anterior wall of the left ventricle.

(B) The left circumflex artery supplies blood to the lateral and posterior walls of the left ventricle.

(C) The right coronary artery supplies blood to the inferior wall of the left ventricle.

(D) The left main coronary artery supplies blood to the apex of the left ventricle.

319. Under normal circumstances, which of the following is the correct course of an electrical impulse in the conduction system of the heart?

(A) atrioventricular (AV) node, sino-atrial (SA) node, bundle of His, internodal atrial pathways, right and left bundle branches, Purkinje fibers, ventricular muscle

(B) bundle of His, SA node, ventricular muscle, AV node, internodal atrial pathways, right and left bundle branches, Purkinje fibers

(C) SA node, Purkinje fibers, AV node, right and left bundle branches, ventricular muscle, bundle of His, internodal atrial pathways

(D) SA node, internodal atrial pathways, AV node, bundle of His, right and left bundle branches, Purkinje fibers, ventricular muscle

320. All of the following are correct statements concerning some of the pacemaker sites in the heart EXCEPT

(A) The AV node is normally the dominant pacemaker in the heart.

(B) If the SA node is damaged or not functioning properly and the AV node becomes the pacemaker for the heart, the heart rate is usually 40 to 60 beats per minute.

(C) If the ventricle or Purkinje fibers become the pacemaker for the heart, the heart rate is usually 20 to 40 beats per minute.

(D) The SA node paces the heart normally at 60 to 100 beats per minute.

321. All of the following are stages of cardiac muscle excitation EXCEPT

(A) polarization

(B) depolarization

(C) repolarization

(D) deportation

322. Electrolytes play a key role in the myocardial action potential. All of the following are such electrolytes, listed with their functions, EXCEPT

(A) phosphorus (P): involved in the depolarization of the myocardial cells

(B) sodium (Na): plays a major role in depolarization of the myocardium

(C) calcium (Ca): plays a role in myocardial depolarization and contraction

(D) potassium (K): plays a major role in repolarization of the myocardium

323. Starling's law of the heart is defined as

(A) The pressure in the left ventricle of the heart is proportional to the pressure in the right ventricle.

(B) The stroke volume of the heart is directly related to the diastolic pressure.

(C) The more the myocardium is stretched, up to a limit, the greater its force of contraction.

(D) The myocardial resting pressure is directly proportional to the inverse of the systolic blood pressure.

324. All of the following are parts of the autonomic nervous system EXCEPT

    (A) parasympathetic system
    (B) the vagus nerve
    (C) nervous stomach
    (D) the sympathetic system

325. All of the following are effects of the various parts of the autonomic nervous system on the heart EXCEPT

    (A) The parasympathetic system slows the heart rate and increases myocardial contractility.
    (B) The sympathetic nervous system increases the heart rate and increases myocardial contractility.
    (C) The sympathetic beta-receptor stimulation produces bronchodilation.
    (D) The sympathetic alpha-receptor stimulation produces peripheral vasoconstriction.

326. Match the following pathophysiologies with the list of cardiac diseases:

    (A) angina pectoris _____
    (B) acute pulmonary edema _____
    (C) right ventricular heart failure

    _____
    (D) cardiac arrest _____
    (E) acute myocardial infarction

    _____
    (F) dissecting aortic aneurysm

    _____
    (G) deep venous thrombosis _____
    (H) acute pulmonary emboli _____

    1. thrombus or clot in an atherosclerotic coronary artery
    2. common causes are left ventricular congestive heart failure, COPD, and pulmonary emboli
    3. most severe form of left ventricular congestive heart failure
    4. believed to be caused by a lethal dysrhythmia
    5. small tear in the inner wall of the aorta
    6. caused by air, fat, amniotic fluid, or blood clots
    7. commonly caused by atherosclerosis and spasm
    8. blood clot in the veins

327. All of the following are signs of cardiovascular disease that can be detected by careful inspection of the patient EXCEPT

    (A) skin color and capillary refill
    (B) jugular vein distention
    (C) facial rash
    (D) peripheral edema

328. All of the following are physical findings that are detectable by auscultation EXCEPT

(A) carotid bruits
(B) lung sounds
(C) abdominal tenderness
(D) heart sounds

329. All of the following are signs of cardiovascular disease that can be detected by palpation EXCEPT

(A) weak, thready pulse
(B) rapid pulse rate
(C) asymmetrical pulses
(D) distant heart sounds

330. All of the following are correct statements about heart sounds EXCEPT

(A) The first heart sound, known as S_1, is produced by the venous return blood entering the right atrium.
(B) The second heart sound, known as S_2, is produced by the closure of the aortic and pulmonic valves.
(C) The third heart sound, known as S_3, is associated with congestive heart failure and is a pathologic heart sound.
(D) The fourth heart sound, known as S_4, is produced by left and right atrial contraction.

331. In obtaining a focused history for the patient with a cardiovascular emergency, all of the following are important EXCEPT

(A) chief complaint
(B) present illness: history of the present event
(C) review of systems: genitourinary, gastrointestinal, neurologic, and so on
(D) significant past medical history

332. The purpose of ECG monitoring is to determine the

(A) myocardial contractile capability
(B) oxygen saturation in the blood
(C) presence of left ventricular hypertrophy
(D) presence and type of electrical activity of the heart

333. Match the following ECG waves with the correct cardiac electrical event.

(A) P wave _____
(B) P-R interval _____
(C) T wave _____
(D) QRS _____
(E) R-R interval _____
(F) S-T segment _____

1. ventricular repolarization
2. time between two ventricular depolarizations
3. atrial depolarization
4. atrial depolarization plus AV junction delay
5. time between ventricular depolarization and repolarization
6. ventricular depolarization

334. Match the following electrical events with the correct time intervals.

(A) P-R interval _____
(B) junctional rhythm _____
(C) QRS interval _____
(D) normal sinus rhythm _____
(E) supraventricular tachycardia
_____
(F) sinus tachycardia _____
_____
(G) sinus bradycardia _____
(H) idioventricular rhythm _____
(I) atrial fibrillation _____
(J) ventricular tachycardia _____

1. 40 to 60 beats per minute
2. 60 to 100 beats per minute
3. 0.12 to 0.20 second
4. 0.08 to 0.12 second
5. 150 to 250 beats per minute
6. atrial rate 350 to 600 per minute
7. lower than 60 beats per minute
8. 100 to 160 beats per minute
9. 20 to 40 beats per minute
10. 100 to 250 beats per minute

335. Match the following ECG leads with the correct area of the heart that they represent.

(A) 2, 3, and AVF _____
(B) tall R waves V_1 and V_2 _____
(C) V_4, V_5, and V_6 _____
(D) V_1, V_2, and V_3 _____

1. anterolateral wall
2. anteroseptal wall
3. inferior wall
4. posterior wall

336. The following rhythm strip represents which of the following cardiac rhythms?

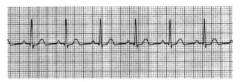

(A) sinus tachycardia
(B) sinus bradycardia
(C) sinus arrest
(D) normal sinus rhythm

337. The following rhythm strip represents which of the following cardiac rhythms?

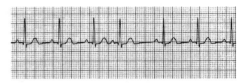

(A) atrial premature contraction
(B) junctional premature contraction
(C) ventricular premature contraction
(D) sinus bradycardia

338. The following rhythm strip represents which of the following cardiac rhythms?

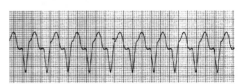

(A) supraventricular tachycardia
(B) ventricular fibrillation
(C) junctional rhythm
(D) ventricular tachycardia

339. The following rhythm strip represents which of the following cardiac rhythms?

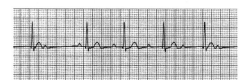

(A) first-degree AV block
(B) second-degree AV block, Mobitz type I
(C) second-degree AV block, Mobitz type II
(D) third-degree AV block

340. The following rhythm strip represents which of the following cardiac rhythms?

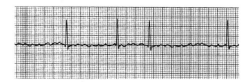

(A) normal sinus rhythm
(B) atrial flutter
(C) atrial fibrillation
(D) supraventricular tachycardia

341. The following rhythm strip represents which of the following cardiac rhythms?

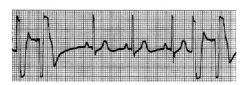

(A) unifocal premature ventricular contraction (PVC)
(B) multifocal PVCs
(C) coupled PVCs
(D) ventricular bigeminy

342. Match the following ECG rhythm strip with the correct dysrhythmia.

1. Multifocal PVCs
2. premature junctional contractions (PJCs)
3. sinus tachycardia
4. ventricular tachycardia

(A) _____

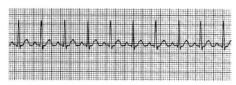

(B) _____

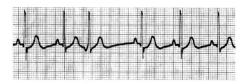

(C) _____

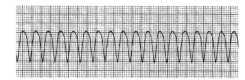

(D) _____

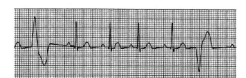

343. Match the following ECG rhythm strips with the correct dysrhythmia.

   1. ventricular fibrillation
   2. junctional rhythm
   3. atrial tachycardia
   4. sinus arrest

(A) _____

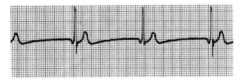

(B) _____

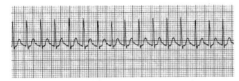

(C) _____

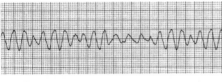

(D) _____

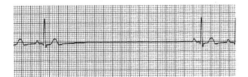

344. Match the following ECG rhythm strips with the correct arrhythmias.

   1. second-degree AV block (Mobitz type I), Wenckebach
   2. unifocal PVCs
   3. accelerated junctional rhythm
   4. second-degree AV block (Mobitz type II), 3:1 AV block

(A) _____

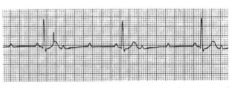

(B) _____

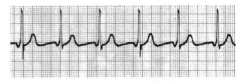

(C) _____

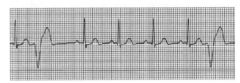

(D) _____

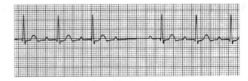

345. Match the following ECG rhythm strips with the correct arrhythmias.

1. atrial flutter
2. third-degree heart block
3. ventricular bigeminy
4. pacemaker rhythm

(A) _____

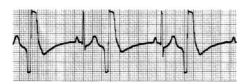

(B) _____

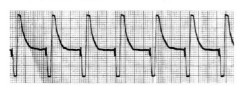

(C) _____

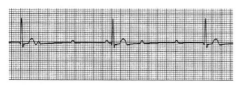

(D) _____

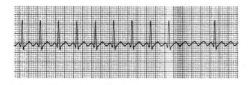

346. All of the following conditions may be associated with pulseless electrical activity (PEA) EXCEPT
(A) cardiogenic shock
(B) anginal syndrome
(C) cardiac tamponade
(D) acute pulmonary embolism

347. All of the following are correct statements concerning the cardiac effects of electrolyte abnormalities EXCEPT

(A) Hypokalemia may produce inverted T waves on the ECG and increases myocardial irritability.
(B) Hypercalcemia may result in increased myocardial contractility.
(C) Hypernatremia may produce ST-segment elevation on the ECG.
(D) Hyperkalemia may result in tall, peaked T waves and cause decreased automaticity and conduction.

348. All of the following are situations in which an ECG rhythm analysis is indicated EXCEPT

(A) patient with chest pain
(B) patient in any form of shock
(C) patient with a very fast or very slow heart rate
(D) patient with a fever

349. Which of the following electrical impulses on the ECG is the most suggestive of acute myocardial ischemia and/or infarction?

(A) P wave
(B) P-R interval
(C) ST segment
(D) T wave

350. You are dispatched to an elderly patient who has passed out at home. Upon arrival at the patient's home, you find an 84-year-male who is lying on the floor. His wife and neighbor were watching the television with the patient and noticed that the patient attempted to walk to the kitchen and suddenly became unconscious and fell to the floor. The patient was unresponsive for 2 to 3 minutes on the floor and upon awakening denied any memory of the event. The patient and witnesses denied any signs suggestive of a seizure, hypoglycemia, headache, palpitations, focal weakness, slurred speech, or a drug ingestion. Initial vital signs revealed that the patient had a blood pressure of 110/68, respirations of 14 per minute, and a pulse of around 70 per minute and irregular. While your partner performed a physical examination, you connected the patient to a cardiac monitor, which revealed the following ECG rhythm strip.

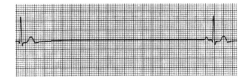

This ECG represents which of the following dysrhythmias?

(A) normal sinus rhythm
(B) sinus tachycardia
(C) sinus bradycardia
(D) sinus arrest

351. Based on the clinical presentation described in question 350, the treatment of choice should be

(A) IV isoproterenol
(B) IV digoxin
(C) IV atropine
(D) IV verapamil

352. You are completing your evaluation and initial treatment of a 68-year-old female with chest pain when you notice that she has suddenly stopped breathing. As you quickly confirm that she is pulseless and unconscious, you quickly check the monitor, which reveals the following dysrhythmia.

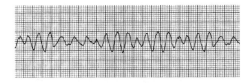

Based upon the above dysrhythmia, the treatment of choice is

(A) IV lidocaine
(B) IV bretylium
(C) immediate defibrillation
(D) synchronized cardioversion

353. As you begin to defibrillate the patient with 200 joules, then 300 joules, and finally 360 joules, the patient continues to remain in ventricular fibrillation. All of the following are part of the emergent treatment of the patient who remains in ventricular defibrillation after initially unsuccessful defibrillation EXCEPT

(A) IV lidocaine and bretylium
(B) endotracheal intubation
(C) IV calcium
(D) IV epinephrine

354. You are dispatched to a " sick patient." As you arrive at the patient's home, you find a 48-year-old male who admits to having substernal chest pain, shortness of breath, sweating, and nausea for the past 2 hours. Upon further questioning, the patient admits to smoking 2 packs of cigarettes per day for the past 30 years, to having been on medication for high blood pressure for the past 5 years, and that his father died of an acute heart attack at age 45. Your partner took the patient's vital signs and found the patient breathing at 26 times per minute, with a blood pressure of 148/72 and a regular pulse rate of 130 per minute. The patient's primary assessment is grossly normal. Your partner has hooked the patient up to a cardiac monitor and presents you with the following ECG rhythm strip.

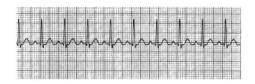

Based upon your interpretation of the ECG, the correct initial treatment is

(A) IV digoxin
(B) sublingual nitroglycerin
(C) IV diltiazem
(D) IV lidocaine

355. As you begin to transport the patient, your patient begins to complain of a funny heartbeat. As you inspect the monitor, you find the patient in the following rhythm.

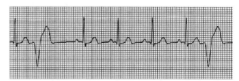

Based upon your interpretation of this ECG rhythm strip, after administering oxygen, the treatment of choice is which of the following?

(A) IV lidocaine
(B) IV bretylium
(C) IV atropine
(D) analgesics for his chest pain

356. You are dispatched to a skilled nursing facility to evaluate and transport a 94-year-old male resident who complains of nausea and vomiting associated with dizziness and feeling a little weak. The patient's vital signs are blood pressure 100/70, respirations 16 per minute, and pulse 54 per minute. The patient's initial assessment reveals a 94-year-old male, awake, weak, and in no acute distress. As you begin to apply oxygen by nonrebreather face mask, you connect the patient to an ECG monitor, which reveals the following rhythm.

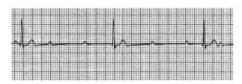

Based upon this rhythm, the treatment of choice, with medical control approval, is which of the following?

(A) IV atropine
(B) IV diltiazem
(C) sublingual nitroglycerin
(D) transcutaneous pacing

357. As you arrive at the scene of a suspected drug overdose on a Friday night in the back of a schoolyard, you notice a group of nine teenagers. One of the bystanders begins to tell you that this young 16-year-old male had been told today that his girlfriend was breaking up with him. He supposedly ran home and gathered up some of his father's medications and ingested a whole bottle of blood pressure pills of unknown type. As your partner has already begun to assess the patient, he notes that the patient has stopped breathing. Initially, a quick look with the monitor-defibrillator paddles reveals that the patient is in the rhythm below. Since you have confirmed that he is pulseless and apneic, you begin CPR, prepare to perform endotracheal intubation with 100 percent oxygen, connect to a cardiac monitor, and begin an IV line.

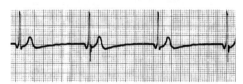

Based upon this rhythm and the patient's clinical presentation the initial treatment of choice is

(A) IV lidocaine
(B) SC epinephrine
(C) IV atropine 1.0 mg
(D) IV epinephrine 1.0 mg

358. As you continue to treat the patient in cardiac arrest described in question 357, you are becoming frustrated because, despite your best efforts, the patient remains in the same heart rhythm, in PEA. While you have frantically searched for treatable causes of PEA, a friend of the patient has retrieved the empty vile of medications from the patient's home, Cardizem CD 240 mg tablets, dated yesterday, with 90 tablets. Now you immediately begin to package the patient for transport, because you realize that this patient's PEA may be corrected with which of the following medications, which you do not carry in your medication box and is readily available in all emergency departments?

(A) IV digoxin
(B) IV Solumedrol
(C) IV Narcan
(D) IV calcium

359. As you arrive at the scene of a motor vehicle accident, you find a 23-year-old female sitting in the back seat of a taxicab who is complaining of being upset but denies any focal pain, headache, whiplash, arm tingling, or numbness. An examination of the vehicle reveals minimal dents on the front bumper and the front left headlight. Upon initial assessment, the patient appears to show no evidence of any trauma, with vital signs as follows: blood pressure 104/68, respirations 14 per minute, and pulse 44 per minute. Upon further questioning, the patient denies taking any medications, drug ingestion, nausea or vomiting, and so on. However, the patient does admit to running 5 miles per day and has been noted to have a slow pulse. As you connect the patient to a cardiac monitor, the patient has the following ECG strip.

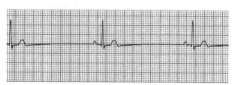

Based upon this ECG and this clinical presentation, which of the following is the correct course of treatment?

(A) IV atropine
(B) IV isoproterenol
(C) repeat vital signs and secondary assessment
(D) transcutaneous pacing

360. All of the following are indications for the use of transcutaneous pacing EXCEPT

    (A) symptomatic sinus bradycardia
    (B) symptomatic atrial fibrillation with a slow ventricular rate
    (C) third-degree heart block with a slow ventricular rate
    (D) ventricular fibrillation

361. You arrive at the home of an 86-year-old male who was found unconscious sitting in his favorite chair, for an unknown period of time. His wife had gone to the store 3 hours ago and left him reading the morning newspaper. As you immediately place the patient on the floor, you realize that he is not breathing and is pulseless. Your partner immediately connects the patient to an ECG monitor, which reveals the following rhythm.

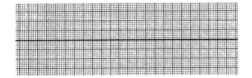

Based upon this rhythm, the correct choice of treatment is which of the following

    (A) immediate defibrillation
    (B) CPR, intubate, IV access, confirm in more than 1 lead
    (C) IV lidocaine
    (D) IV bretylium

362. All of the following are parts of the process of treating a patient with a transcutaneous pacemaker EXCEPT

    (A) Explain the procedure to the patient, place the patient in an upright position, and administer oxygen, IV line, and ECG monitoring.
    (B) Confirm the presence of an indication for pacing, such as symptomatic bradycardia, and medical control approval.
    (C) Apply the pacing electrodes, connect them to the pacemaker cable, and set the desired pacer rate at 60 to 80 beats per minute.
    (D) Set voltage at 0, turn the pacer on, and slowly increase the voltage until ventricular capture.

363. All of the following are ECG rhythm strip signs of pacemaker malfunction EXCEPT

    (A) slow heart rate, less than 60 to 70 per minute, without pacemaker spike activity
    (B) pacemaker spikes without QRS complex following
    (C) heart rhythm over 90 per minute without pacemaker spikes
    (D) pacemaker spikes firing on top of or after the QRS complex

364. Which of the following is the most common cause of pacemaker failure?

    (A) battery failure
    (B) hypoglycemia
    (C) infection
    (D) electrolyte imbalance

365. All of the following are risk factors for coronary artery disease with the development of angina pectoris or myocardial infarction EXCEPT

(A) cigarette smoking
(B) hypertension
(C) hypercholesterolemia
(D) family history of peptic ulcer disease

366. You arrive at the scene of a 64-year-old male who was carrying garbage cans to the street when he suddenly developed substernal chest pain, sweating, difficulty breathing, and nausea, and actually was so weak that he sat down on the grass. As you begin to treat and continue to assess this patient, you think about the pathophysiology of angina pectoris. Which of the following is the best explanation?

(A) blockage of all coronary arteries, with no coronary artery blood supply to the heart
(B) all coronary arteries in spasm, resulting in lack of oxygen to the heart
(C) increased myocardial oxygen requirements due to increased exertion, and insufficient myocardial oxygen supply due to coronary artery disease
(D) partial blockage of coronary arteries, resulting in increased demands of oxygen

367. The most common ECG finding in angina pectoris is
(A) ST-segment depression
(B) PR-interval prolongation
(C) tall, peaked T waves
(D) Q waves

368. In approaching the patient with angina pectoris, which of the following is the correct description of the treatment of this patient?

(A) Assume that angina is not a myocardial infarction and treat accordingly.
(B) With a clinical presentation consistent with ischemic chest pain, assume that the patient may be having an acute myocardial infarction and treat accordingly.
(C) Before treating this patient, begin to question intensely in order to select a treatment path for an acute myocardial infarction or angina.
(D) If you are unsure whether the patient is suffering from angina or an acute myocardial infarction, refrain from any treatment and transport.

369. You are driving back to your garage when a woman who claims that her sister is having a heart attack frantically waves you down. As you walk up three flights of stairs, you find a 58-year-old female sitting in a chair. She is pale and breathing at 32 times per minute. As the patient begins to tell of her severe chest pain radiating down her left arm, your partner begins to initiate emergent treatment of the patient. This will include all of the following EXCEPT

(A) Administer 100% oxygen by non-rebreather face mask.
(B) Attach to an ECG monitor.
(C) Perform a 12-lead ECG immediately, as the first intervention.
(D) Administer a sublingual nitroglycerin 0.4-mg tablet.

370. As you continue to provide emergent prehospital care to the patient described in question 369, you begin to think of the possible complications of an acute myocardial infarction. All of the following are possible complications of an acute myocardial infarction EXCEPT

(A) lethal cardiac dysrhythmias
(B) brain tumor
(C) cardiogenic shock
(D) cardiac rupture

371. All of the following are correct statements concerning an acute myocardial infarction EXCEPT

(A) Sixty to 70 percent occur outside the hospital.
(B) They are responsible for 500,000 deaths per year in the United States.
(C) They are the leading cause of death in the United States.
(D) Five to 7 percent of patients have no pain.

372. All of the following are hemodynamic changes associated with an acute myocardial infarction EXCEPT

(A) normal blood pressure
(B) high blood pressure
(C) low blood pressure
(D) increased respiratory rate

373. As you arrive at a factory for a patient with chest pain, you find a 48-year-old male who appears diaphoretic, pale, clammy, and short of breath. Upon questioning, the patient admits to an acute onset of substernal chest pain, described as a squeezing-type pain, which has gradually worsened. The patient was lifting several heavy boxes at the time of the incident. He also admitted to smoking three packs of cigarettes a day, high blood pressure, and an elevated cholesterol level. He also noted that his father had a heart attack at 35 years of age. As you begin to assess and treat this patient with a possible acute myocardial infarction, you focus upon the parameters that you need to assess. All of the following are items to be assessed EXCEPT

(A) ECG monitoring
(B) repeat vital signs
(C) skin turgor
(D) repeat lung sounds

374. All of the following are evolutionary ECG changes associated with an acute myocardial infarction EXCEPT

(A) ST-segment depression
(B) T-wave inversion
(C) P-wave inversion
(D) ST-segment elevation

375. You are in the midst of treating a patient at a school fair for a minor allergic reaction when one of the workers asks you to come and evaluate a man with chest pain. The new patient is a 54-year-old male who has been carrying heavy beer barrels into the fairgrounds for the past hour and has suddenly developed substernal chest pain about 20 minutes ago. The patient describes the pain as like "someone sitting on my chest" and admits that the pain radiates down both arms and is associated with palpitations, weakness, and profuse sweating. He also admits to being under a doctor's care for high blood pressure, diabetes, and poor circulation in his legs. As you begin to assess and treat this patient, you begin to think about him as a possible candidate for thrombolytic therapy. All of the following are inclusion criteria for thrombolytic therapy EXCEPT

(A) age over 40 years
(B) pain not relieved by nitroglycerin
(C) ST-segment elevation over 1 mm in two adjacent leads
(D) chest pain for longer than 20 minutes and less than 6 hours

376. You are sent to a construction site for a 10-foot fall from a scaffold. As you arrive at the patient's side, the story becomes a little more complicated. The 58-year-old male patient states that he slipped off the scaffold 20 minutes ago. He states that he is having severe pain in his right ankle and mid-chest. He admits to being treated for angina for 2 years and now complains about the chest pain becoming more intense, despite taking a nitroglycerin tablet about 5 minutes ago. As you begin to complete a primary assessment on this patient, you are contemplating the possibility of this patient's becoming a candidate for thrombolytic therapy. After quickly assessing the patient's chest and confirming that there is no gross evidence of chest trauma, rib fractures, pneumothorax, or chest wounds, you administer another nitroglycerin tablet without relief. A quick examination of his right ankle reveals a grossly deformed, angulated fracture, with a large pool of blood surrounding it. This patient would be excluded from being treated with thrombolytic therapy because of which of the following exclusion criteria?

(A) age
(B) terminal illness
(C) significant bleeding
(D) gastrointestinal or genitourinary bleeding

377. Match the following drugs with the common dose and therapeutic effect.

(A) atropine sulfate _____
(B) procainamide _____
(C) morphine sulfate _____
(D) dopamine _____
(E) furosemide _____
(F) adenosine _____
(G) verapamil _____
(H) lidocaine _____

1. 1 to 1.5 mg/kg IV; suppress ventricular dysrhythmias
2. 6 mg IV bolus; terminate supraventricular tachycardia
3. 0.5 mg IV bolus; parasympatholytic agent
4. 3 to 5 mg slow IV push; pain relief and venodilation
5. 20 to 40 mg IV push; venodilation and diuresis
6. 20 to 30 mg/kg IV; ventricular dysrhythmias resistant to lidocaine
7. 2.5 to 20 mcg/kg/min; vasopressor
8. 2.5 to 5 mg IV bolus; terminate supraventricular tachycardia

378. Match the following cardiovascular drugs with the correct side effects.

(A) nitrates _____
(B) beta blockers _____
(C) calcium blockers _____
(D) isoproterenol _____
(E) furosemide _____

1. hypotension
2. hypokalemia
3. bradycardia
4. increased heart rate and myocardial contractility
5. headache and tingling under the tongue

379. All of the following are causes of left ventricular heart failure EXCEPT

(A) acute myocardial infarction
(B) valvular heart disease
(C) chronic hypertension
(D) advanced COPD

380. All of the following are symptoms of left ventricular heart failure EXCEPT

(A) dyspnea
(B) paroxysmal nocturnal dyspnea
(C) orthopnea
(D) headache

381. You are dispatched to a "difficulty breathing" patient. As you enter the patient's home, you find a 76-year-old female sitting up in bed with three pillows behind her back. The patient tells you that she has had similar episodes in the past because of a very large heart, believed to be due to high blood pressure and two previous myocardial infarctions. As your partner begins to administer oxygen, you begin to perform an initial assessment of this patient with acute pulmonary edema. You would expect to observe all of the following physical findings EXCEPT

(A) diffuse, moist rales in the lungs
(B) absent pulses
(C) neck vein distention
(D) pink, frothy sputum

382. All of the following are possible causes of precipitating acute pulmonary edema EXCEPT

(A) acute myocardial infarction
(B) strep throat
(C) dysrhythmias
(D) acute endocarditis

383. You are dispatched to a nearby nursing home because of an elderly resident complaining of acute difficulty breathing. As you arrive at the patient's bedside, you find a 90-year-old female breathing at 44 respirations per minute. The patient's nurse states that the patient has a history of congestive heart failure for the past 2 years and has been maintained on digoxin, lasix, and periodic nasal oxygen. The patient is in the nursing home because of a long-term history of dementia and has been bed bound for the past 3 months. As you begin to examine the patient, you find a blood pressure of 210/104, a pulse of 120 and regular, and that the patient is afebrile, with jugular neck vein distention and bilateral moist rales throughout the entire chest. All of the following are parts of the treatment of this patient EXCEPT

(A) 100 percent oxygen by non-rebreather face mask
(B) nitroglycerin 0.4 mg tablet
(C) furosemide 5 mg IV bolus
(D) morphine sulfate 2 to 3 mg slow IV

384. The main therapeutic action of morphine sulfate, which results in improvement in the pulmonary edema patient, is which of the following?

(A) alleviates anxiety
(B) slows heart rate
(C) lowers blood pressure
(D) decreases venous return (preload)

385. Which of the following is the best definition of *cardiac tamponade*?

(A) As blood fills the pericardial sac, the coronary arteries become occluded.
(B) As blood fills the ventricles, the aortic and mitral valves fail.
(C) As blood fills the pericardium, the blood pressure elevates dramatically.
(D) As blood fills the pericardium, the heart's function is progressively compromised.

386. You are dispatched to a shooting at the scene of a robbery. As you pull up to the store, you find a 30-year-old male lying unconscious on the floor. As you begin to assess the patient, you notice that he has a blood-stained shirt. His airway is patent, and he is breathing at 22 breaths per minute, has a pulse rate of 130 per minute, and has a blood pressure only palpable at 50 systolic. Upon further examination, the patient's lung sounds are clear and symmetrical, he has distended neck veins and cyanosis, and auscultation of the heart reveals crisp heart sounds. All of the following are clinical signs of cardiac tamponade EXCEPT

(A) distended neck veins
(B) hypotension
(C) crisp heart sounds
(D) tachycardia

387. While hypertension is a medical condition that affects over 60 million Americans, the definition of a hypertensive emergency includes an acute elevation of blood pressure along with evidence of end-organ damage. All of the following are examples of end-organ damage, which is caused by uncontrolled hypertension, EXCEPT

(A) cancer
(B) acute pulmonary edema
(C) dissecting aortic aneurysm
(D) hypertensive encephalopathy

388. You arrive at the home of a 56-year-old male whose wife states that he had initially been acting confused since lunch but now has become increasingly sleepy and difficult to arouse. She states that he does not drink alcohol and does not take any medications. He had been told he had high blood pressure, and his physician had started him on blood pressure medications a year ago, but he did not continue to take them and has not seen his physician again. He had been complaining of a headache on and off for the past 2 weeks and was taking more aspirin and Tylenol than usual. Upon examining the patient, you notice that he is breathing at 20 respirations per minute, with a pulse of 84 per minute and a bood pressure of 240/130 bilaterally. The patient's entire physical assessment is grossly normal, without any signs of focal weakness. As you contemplate an approach to treatment of this patient with a hypertensive emergency, you consider administering all of the following treatment options, with medical control approval, EXCEPT

(A) dilantin 500 mg IV push
(B) furosemide 20 to 40 mg IV push
(C) nitroglycerin 0.4 mg sublingual tablet or spray
(D) nifedipine 10 mg capsule, punctured and released under the patient's tongue

389. All of the following are signs of cardiogenic shock EXCEPT

(A) cool, clammy skin
(B) tachypnea
(C) hypertension
(D) tachycardia

390. You arrive at the scene of a chest-pain patient and find a 68-year-old male patient lying on the floor, diaphoretic, and breathing at 40 breaths per minute. He is cool and clammy, has a pulse of 130 beats per minute, and appears very weak and lethargic. The patient is unable to give a history, and his blood pressure is only 40 systolic palpable bilaterally. As your partner begins to apply oxygen, connect to an ECG monitor, and initiate an IV line, the patient's wife states that he has had two previous myocardial infarctions, suffers from congestive heart failure, and complained of substernal chest pain this morning for 25 minutes prior to the call to 911. As you complete your assessment of the patient, you contemplate treatment options. Which of the following would appear to be the best initial treatment of this patient?

(A) norepinephrine (Levophed) 0.5 to 30 μg/min
(B) digoxin 1.0 mg IV slowly over 2 minutes
(C) pneumatic antishock trousers
(D) dopamine (Intropin), initially 2 to 5 μg/kg/min

391. All of the following are acute emergencies that may progress to cardiac arrest EXCEPT

(A) acute myocardial infarction
(B) viral flu syndrome
(C) foreign-body airway obstruction
(D) drowning

392. All of the following are the most common conditions associated with the cardiac arrest patient EXCEPT

(A) first-degree heart block
(B) ventricular fibrillation
(C) asystole
(D) pulseless electrical activity

393. You are dispatched to a hardware store for a 50-year-old unconscious patient. However, when you arrive and begin to examine the patient, you note that she is unresponsive, pulseless, and apneic. You immediately reach for which of the following piece of equipment?

(A) oxygen mask
(B) IV line
(C) nitroglycerin tablet
(D) quick-look monitor-defibrillator paddles

394. As you respond to a cardiac arrest call, you find a 76-year-old female lying in the hallway of an apartment building. The patient is unresponsive, pulseless, and apneic. As you begin to perform a quick-look with the ECG monitor paddles, you find that the patient is in a junctional tachycardia. Rechecking, you find that the patient is truly without a pulse. As you begin to perform CPR, you try to reflect on the possible correctable causes of pulseless electrical activity (PEA). All of the following are possible correctable causes of PEA EXCEPT

(A) hyperventilation
(B) tension pneumothorax
(C) cardiac tamponade
(D) severe hypovolemia

395. Match each of the following medications, which are used in treating cardiac arrest patients, with the correct desired therapeutic effect.

(A) IV lidocaine _____
(B) IV epinephrine _____
(C) IV atropine _____
(D) IV magnesium sulfate _____
(E) IV sodium bicarbonate _____
(F) IV bretylium tosylate _____

1. corrects metabolic acidosis
2. increases cerebral and coronary blood flow
3. prevents recurrence of ventricular fibrillation
4. corrects magnesium deficiency
5. prevents recurrence of ventricular tachycardia
6. may stimulate activity in asystole

396. All of the following are critical actions required for treating patients in nontraumatic cardiac arrest EXCEPT

(A) administering IV calcium
(B) applying quick-look ECG monitor-defibrillator
(C) starting IV access
(D) endotracheal intubation

397. All of the following are criteria for termination of resuscitation EXCEPT

(A) standard advanced cardiac life support for 25 minutes
(B) no restoration of spontaneous circulation
(C) absence of recurring or refractory ventricular fibrillation or ventricular tachycardia or continued neurologic activity
(D) patient's family is upset with resuscitation efforts

398. You are sent to a 64-year-old male with acute nontraumatic leg pain. As you arrive at the patient's bedside, you find the patient grimacing in pain, pointing to his left leg. The patient admits to smoking three packs of cigarettes per day and has a history of mild diabetes but again denies any recent trauma. Upon examination, you find the patient's left leg to be pale, cool, cyanotic, and pulseless, and the patient has decreased ability to move his left foot. This patient's presentation is consistent with which of the following diagnoses?

(A) acute phlebitis
(B) acute cellulitis
(C) acute arterial occlusion
(D) acute arthritis

399. Which of the following cardiac dysrhythmias would be one of the possible causes of the patient's emergent problem in question 398?

(A) ventricular tachycardia
(B) atrial fibrillation
(C) sinus rhythm
(D) junctional tachycardia

400. Which of the following is the correct definition of *aneurysm*?

(A) blockage of an artery
(B) pulsating narrowing of a vessel
(C) congenital defect of a vein
(D) weakening and dilation of a vessel wall

401. *Claudication* is defined as

(A) acute swelling of the chest wall
(B) intermittent heat and redness of a leg
(C) cramplike pain in the calf
(D) focal headache

402. All of the following are types of aneurysms EXCEPT

(A) atherosclerotic
(B) congenital
(C) traumatic
(D) embolic

403. You are dispatched to the scene of a chest-pain patient. As you walk into the office, you find a 65-year-old male lying on the office floor. He states that he has substernal chest pain, which began 1 hour ago and has a ripping quality. He states that the pain was very severe at onset and remains the same but now is moving from the substernal location to the epigastric area. In taking the patient's vital signs, your partner is confused because he found the blood pressure to be 178/68 in the right arm and 120/52 in the left arm, even with repeating the readings twice. This patient's presentation is most suggestive of

(A) dissecting aortic aneurysm
(B) acute myocardial infarction
(C) acute arterial occlusion
(D) peptic ulcer disease

404. While on your way for gas, a bystander, who states that her father is having severe stomach pains that spread to his back, flags you down. As you gather your equipment, you have found out that the patient is a 70-year-old male who has had acute abdominal pain for only 30 minutes, and it was not associated with vomiting, diarrhea, or fever. As you arrive at the patient's bedside, you find an acutely ill, pale patient who appears to be writhing in pain. As you begin to examine the patient, you find that the patient has a blood pressure of 50 palpable bilaterally, no bowel sounds, and a pulsating abdominal mass. This patient appears to have which of the following acute emergencies?

(A) acute appendicitis
(B) acute low back strain
(C) acute urinary retention
(D) acute abdominal aortic aneurysm

405. All of the following are parts of the prehospital emergency medical care for a patient with an abdominal aortic aneurysm EXCEPT

(A) high-concentration oxygen
(B) ECG monitoring
(C) IV access
(D) on-scene stabilization if the patient is hypotensive

406. As you transport a 64-year-old female patient with possibly her third acute myocardial infarction, her emotionally upset daughter asks you if there is anything that she may do in order to prevent heart disease for herself and her children. Before you answer, you begin to think of the risk factors for cardiovascular disease that can be modified. All of the following are modifiable risk factors EXCEPT

(A) hypertension
(B) family history of premature cardiovascular disease
(C) smoking
(D) hypercholesterolemia

MEDICAL CARDIOLOGY

ANSWERS

313. The answer is B. (Mosby, *Cardiovascular Emergencies*; Brady, *Cardiovascular Emergencies*.) (A), (C), and (D) are correct statements. (B) is an incorrect statement because approximately 50 percent of deaths from cardiovascular diseases are believed to be due to myocardial infarctions.

314. The answer is A. (Mosby, *Cardiovascular Emergencies*.) (B), (C), (D), diabetes, age, obesity, male sex, and a family history of premature coronary artery disease are all major risk factors for coronary artery disease. (A) is incorrect because cigarette smoking by the individual, not a history of smoking by a family member, is a major risk factor.

315. The answer is A. (Caroline/Little Brown, *Cardiovascular Emergencies*.) (B), (C), and (D) are correct statements. (A) is an incorrect statement because the heart is located above the diaphragm, posterior to and slightly to the left of the sternum.

316. The answer is C. (Caroline/Little Brown, *Cardiovascular Emergencies*.) (C) is the correct sequence in following the flow of blood from the left ventricle to all of the body by way of the arterial system and then returning by way of the venous system. (A), (B), and (D) are all incorrect.

317. The answer is C. (Brady, *Cardiovascular Emergencies*.) (C) is the correct formula used to determine cardiac output. (A) is a formula used to show the relationship between blood pressure and cardiac output and peripheral resistance. (B) is Einstein's famous formula for determining energy. (D) is incorrect.

318. **The answer is D.** (Brady, *Cardiovascular Emergencies.*) (A), (B), and (C) are all correct examples. (D) is an incorrect example because the left main coronary artery supplies blood to its branches, the left anterior descending (LAD) artery, and the left circumflex artery. While the left main coronary artery normally supplies all of the coronary artery blood supply to its two branches, it is usually not associated with supplying blood to any particular geographic area of the left ventricle.

319. **The answer is D.** (Brady, *Cardiovascular Emergencies.*) (D) is the correct sequence for an electrical impulse to follow in the normal heart. (A), (B), and (C) are incorrect.

320. **The answer is A.** (Mosby, *Cardiovascular Emergencies.*) (B), (C), and (D) are correct statements. (A) is not a correct statement because the SA node is normally the dominant pacemaker in the heart.

321. **The answer is D.** (Brady, *Cardiovascular Emergencies.*) (A), (B), and (C) are all stages of cardiac muscle excitation. (D) is unrelated to cardiac muscle excitation. It refers to being banished from a country.

322. **The answer is A.** (Brady, *Cardiovascular Emergencies.*) (B), (C), and (D) are all involved in the myocardial action potential. (A) is the exception because phosphorus (P), while a very important electrolyte in the body, is not involved in the myocardial action potential.

323. **The answer is C.** (Brady, *Cardiovascular Emergencies.*) (A), (B), and (D) are incorrect. (C) is correct because the greater the volume of blood filling the chamber, the more forceful the myocardial contraction. Therefore, the greater the venous return, the greater the preload, and the greater the stroke volume.

324. **The answer is C.** (Caroline/Little Brown, *Cardiovascular Emergencies.*) (A), (B), and (D) are all parts of the autonomic nervous system. (C) is the exception because a nervous stomach is usually a symptom of anxiety or stress, but not a part of the nervous system.

325. **The answer is A.** (Mosby, *Cardiovascular Emergencies.*) (B), (C), and (D) are correct statements. (A) is an incorrect statement because, while the parasympathetic nervous system slows the heart rate, it also decreases myocardial contractility.

326. **Answers.** (Brady, *Cardiovascular Emergencies.*)
   (A) 7
   (B) 3
   (C) 2
   (D) 4
   (E) 1
   (F) 5
   (G) 8
   (H) 6

327. **The answer is C.** (Brady, *Cardiovascular Emergencies.*) (A), (B), and (D) may all be signs of cardiovascular disease. (C) is the exception because a facial rash usually is not a sign of cardiovascular disease.

328. **The answer is C.** (Brady, *Cardiovascular Emergencies.*) (A), (B), and (D) are all findings detectable by auscultation. (C) is the exception because abdominal tenderness is detected by palpation of the abdomen, not auscultation.

329. **The answer is D.** (Brady, *Cardiovascular Emergencies.*) (A), (B), and (C) are correct. (D) is incorrect because distant heart sounds are detected by auscultation of the heart, not by palpation.

330. **The answer is A.** (Brady, *Cardiovascular Emergencies.*) (B), (C), and (D) are correct. (A) is incorrect because the first heart sound is produced by the closure of the tricuspid and mitral AV valves.

331. **The answer is C.** (Mosby, *Cardiovascular Emergencies.*) (A), (B), and (D) are correct. (C) is incorrect because the review of systems, while being a part of a complete history and physical examination, is not a part of a focused history in a patient with a cardiovascular emergency. The review of systems would be taken at the emergency department, after the patient is stabilized.

332. **The answer is D.** (Brady, *Cardiovascular Emergencies.*) (D) is correct. (A) is incorrect because the ECG does not give any information about the myocardial muscle contracting capability; an echocardiogram would determine myocardial muscle contractility. Pulse oximetry, not ECG monitoring, determines the oxygen saturation (B). Left and right ventricular hypertrophy (C) is determined by a 12-lead ECG or by an echocardiogram, not by ECG monitoring.

333. **Answers.** (Caroline/Little Brown. *Cardiovascular Emergencies.*)
 (A) 3
 (B) 4
 (C) 1
 (D) 6
 (E) 2
 (F) 5

334. **Answers.** (Caroline/Little Brown, *Cardiovascular Emergencies*; Mosby, *Cardiovascular Emergencies.*)
 (A) 3 (F) 8
 (B) 1 (G) 7
 (C) 4 (H) 9
 (D) 2 (I) 6
 (E) 5 (J) 10

335. **Answers.** (Caroline/Little Brown, *Cardiovascular Emergencies.*)
  (A) 3
  (B) 4
  (C) 1
  (D) 2

336. **The answer is D.** (Caroline/Little Brown, *Cardiovascular Emergencies.*) (D) Normal sinus rhythm is a regular rhythm, with P waves before every QRS complex, at a rate of 60 to 100 beats per minute. (A) is incorrect because sinus tachycardia has a rate of 100 to 160 beats per minute. (B) is incorrect because sinus bradycardia has a rate of less than 60 beats per minute. (C) is incorrect because sinus arrest has a period of no electrical activity (pause), which is not demonstrated here.

337. **The answer is A.** (Caroline/Little Brown, *Cardiovascular Emergencies.*) (A) is correct because there is a premature P wave, which is different from the normal P wave. (B) is incorrect because, with junctional premature contraction, there is a premature QRS complex, which may have no P wave. If a P wave is present, it comes either shortly before (less than 0.12 second) or after the QRS. (C) is incorrect because, with a ventricular premature contraction, the premature QRS is wide (greater than 0.12 second), with a T wave of polarity opposite to that of the QRS. (D) is incorrect because it is a regular rhythm with a rate less than 60 beats per minute.

338. **The answer is D.** (Mosby, *Cardiovascular Emergencies.*) (D) is correct because, with ventricular tachycardia, the rhythm is regular or slightly irregular, with wide QRS complexes (greater than 0.12 second), with a rate of 100 to 250 beats per minute. (A) is incorrect because supraventricular tachycardia usually has narrow QRS complexes (less than 0.12 second) with a regular rhythm and a rate of 150 to 250 beats per minute. (B) is incorrect because ventricular fibrillation is a chaotic, irregular rhythm with no QRS complexes, only fibrillatory waves. (C) is incorrect because a junctional rhythm is a regular rhythm, with narrow QRS complexes and a rate of 40 to 60 beats per minute.

339. **The answer is B.** (Caroline/Little Brown, *Cardiovascular Emergencies.*) (B) is correct because in second-degree AV block, Mobitz type I, also known as Wenckebach, the rhythm is characterized by progressive widening of the P-R interval until an atrial beat is blocked (not followed by a QRS complex). (A) is incorrect, because first-degree AV block is a rhythm characterized by a regular rhythm with a prolonged PR interval greater than 0.20 second). (C) is incorrect, because second-degree AV block, Mobitz type II, is a regular rhythm characterized by P waves not always followed by QRS complexes, with an atrial to ventricular ratio of 2:1, 3:1, 4:1, and so on. (D) is incorrect because third-degree AV block is a regular rhythm characterized by no relationship between the atrial and ventricular complexes, with different rates as well.

340. The answer is C. (Mosby, *Cardiovascular Emergencies.*) (C) is correct because atrial fibrillation is characterized by a rhythm that is irregular, with atrial fibrillatory waves and no P waves. The atrial rate is between 350 to 600 beats per minute, and the ventricular rate is usually between 100 to 160 beats per minute. (A) is incorrect because normal sinus rhythm is characterized by a regular rhythm, with P waves before every QRS, with a rate of 60 to 100 beats per minute. (B) is incorrect because atrial flutter is a regular rhythm with an atrial rate of 250 to 350 beats per minute, with P waves that have the "flutter wave," sawtooth pattern. (D) is incorrect because supraventricular tachycardia is regular and characterized by a regular rhythm with a ventricular rate of 150 to 250 beats per minute.

341. The answer is C. (Caroline/Little Brown, *Cardiovascular Emergencies.*) (C) is correct because coupled PVCs are characterized by premature, wide QRS (greater than 0.12 second), which are repetitive (next to each other). (A) is incorrect because unifocal PVCs are characterized by premature, wide QRS (greater than 0.12 second) from the same focus (appearing the same). (B) is incorrect because multifocal PVCs are characterized by premature, QRS (greater than 0.12 second), which originate in different foci (different appearances). (D) is incorrect because ventricular bigeminy is characterized by a rhythm in which every other beat is a PVC.

342. Answers. (Caroline/Little Brown, *Cardiovascular Emergencies.*)
- (A) 3
- (B) 2
- (C) 4
- (D) 1

343. Answers. (Caroline/Little Brown, *Cardiovascular Emergencies.*)
- (A) 2
- (B) 3
- (C) 1
- (D) 4

344. Answers. (Caroline/Little Brown, *Cardiovascular Emergencies.*)
- (A) 4
- (B) 3
- (C) 2
- (D) 1

345. Answers. (Caroline/Little Brown, *Cardiovascular Emergencies.*)
- (A) 3
- (B) 4
- (C) 2
- (D) 1

346. The answer is B. (Mosby, *Cardiovascular Emergencies*; Brady, *Cardiovascular Emergencies*.) (A), (C), (D), hypovolemia, tension pneumothorax, hypoxemia, acidosis, hyperkalemia, hypothermia, certain drug overdoses (e.g., beta blockers, calcium blockers, tricyclic antidepressants, digoxin, etc.), and any type of shock are all conditions that may be associated with PEA. Ideally, the detection and correction of one of these associated critical conditions may result in the reversal of PEA. (B) is incorrect because patients with anginal syndromes usually have stable vital signs. In PEA, the patient is in cardiac arrest, pulseless, with an electrical rhythm.

347. The answer is C. (Brady, *Cardiovascular Emergencies*.) (A), (B), and (D) are correct. Hypokalemia, a decrease in the blood potassium level, is frequently caused by recurrent vomiting and/or diarrhea and certain potassium-wasting diuretics. Hypercalcemia, an increase in the blood calcium level, is sometimes caused by an excessive intake of calcium tablets, an overactive parathyroid gland, and occasionally with certain types of cancers. Hyperkalemia, an increase in the blood potassium level, is sometimes caused by kidney failure, patients' missing kidney dialysis treatments, metabolic acidosis, and potassium-sparing diuretics. Severe electrolyte imbalances may cause life-threatening dysrhythmias. (C) is incorrect because hypernatremia, an increase in the blood sodium level, does not produce ECG changes. It is most commonly caused by dehydration.

348. The answer is D. (Brady, *Cardiovascular Emergencies*.) (A), (B), (C), and patients suffering from myriad critical and/or potentially unstable conditions, such as cardiac arrest, drug overdose, difficulty breathing, heart failure, major trauma, syncope, coma, anaphylaxis, and so on, are all situations in which an ECG analysis is indicated. (D) is incorrect because a fever by itself is not an indication for ECG rhythm analysis.

349. The answer is C. (Mosby, *Cardiovascular Emergencies*.) (C) is correct because elevation or depression of the ST segment is the most suggestive ECG finding in the patient who may be having acute myocardial ischemia and/or infarction. A series of Q waves in certain parts of the ECG may be evidence of old myocardial infarction(s). (A) is incorrect because the P wave is usually not affected with myocardial ischemia and/or infarction. (B) is incorrect even though, in some acute myocardial infarction patients, one can see prolongation of the P-R interval, known as first-degree heart block. (D) is incorrect even though, in many patients with acute myocardial ischemia and/or infarction, there may be elevation and/or inversion of the T wave. However, a number of abnormalities may affect the T wave, such as an increase or decrease of blood potassium levels, patients' taking digoxin, left ventricular hypertrophy, and bundle-branch blocks.

350. The answer is D. (Brady, *Cardiovascular Emergencies*.) (A), (B), and (C) are incorrect. (D) is correct because there is a long pause of electrical activity before any P-wave activity appears. Significant electrical pauses may be related to a period of loss of consciousness.

351. The answer is C. (Brady, *Cardiovascular Emergencies*.) (C) is correct, with the realization that, if the patient's heart rate fails to respond to the maximal dose of atropine, then the

Paramedic should consider applying a transcutaneous pacemaker. (A), (B), and (D) are incorrect.

352. **The answer is C.** (Mosby, *Cardiovascular Emergencies.*) (C) is the correct immediate treatment for ventricular fibrillation and pulseless ventricular tachycardia. However, in monitored patients who go into ventricular fibrillation or pulseless ventricular tachycardia, performing a precordial thump is also an option. (A), (B), and (D) are incorrect.

353. **The answer is C.** (Mosby, *Cardiovascular Emergencies.*) (A), (B), (D), repeat defibrillation, and possibly sodium bicarbonate are all part of the emergent treatment options available.

354. **The answer is B.** (Mosby, *Cardiovascular Emergencies.*) (B) is correct. Since the ECG rhythm strip is sinus tachycardia with a rate of 130 per minute, there is no treatment for this. The first priority is to treat the patient's chest pain, with medical control approval, with sublingual nitroglycerin. (A), (C), and (D) are all incorrect treatments for sinus tachycardia.

355. **The answer is A.** (Brady, *Cardiovascular Emergencies.*) (A) is correct because the patient is symptomatic with chest pain and malignant PVCs. (B) is incorrect because it is used for more serious ventricular dysrhythmias, such as ventricular fibrillation and ventricular tachycardia, but not for PVCs alone. (C) and (D) are incorrect because neither is the treatment of choice for this patient.

356. **The answer is D.** (Brady, *Cardiovascular Emergencies.*) (D) is correct because, in patients with high-grade heart blocks, atropine (A) should be used with caution, because it may accelerate the atrial rate, while it may worsen the AV nodal block. (B) and (C) are incorrect because they are not part of the treatment of second-degree, Mobitz type II, AV heart block.

357. **The answer is D.** (Caroline/Little Brown, *Cardiovascular Emergencies.*) (D) is the correct answer, since this patient is in cardiac arrest, in the pulseless electrical activity (PEA) algorithm. (A), (B), and (C) are incorrect.

358. **The answer is D.** (Mosby, *Cardiovascular Emergencies.*) (D) is correct because IV calcium is an antidote for any calcium channel blocker overdose. It could potentially return a pulse and blood pressure. (A), (B), and (C) are incorrect.

359. **The answer is C.** (Brady, *Cardiovascular Emergencies.*) (C) is correct because sinus bradycardia is very common in regular long-distance runners. This rhythm should only be treated in patients demonstrating decreased cardiac output, hypotension, angina, or central nervous system symptoms. (A), (B), and (D) are all incorrect in this patient.

360. **The answer is D.** (Mosby, *Cardiovascular Emergencies.*) (A), (B), and (C) may be indications for transcutaneous pacing. (D) is not.

361. **The answer is B.** (Mosby, *Cardiovascular Emergencies.*) (B) is the correct answer, and, after confirming asystole in more than one lead, the next step is the administration of IV epinephrine 1.0 mg, which can be repeated every 3 to 5 minutes. (A), (C), and (D) are incorrect and have no place in the treatment of asystole in the cardiac arrest patient.

362. **The answer is A.** (Brody, *Cardiovascular Emergencies.*) (B), (C), (D), and checking the pulse and blood pressure of the patient are all a part of the process of treating a patient with a transcutaneous pacemaker. (A) is incorrect because you should place the patient in the supine position.

363. **The answer is C.** (Caroline/Little Brown, *Cardiovascular Emergencies.*) (A), (B), and (D) are correct and are examples of ECG manifestations of pacemaker failure. This is true for all types of pacemakers: permanent, temporary transvenous and transcutaneous. (C) is incorrect because, whenever the patient's own heart rate is faster than the rate of the pacemaker, there should be no evidence of pacemaker activity. This pacemaker function is known as sensing.

364. **The answer is A.** (Brady, *Cardiovascular Emergencies.*) (A) is correct. Another cause, in temporary transvenous and permanent pacemakers, is pacemaker lead displacement. (B), (C), and (D) are incorrect.

365. **The answer is D.** (Caroline/Little Brown, *Cardiovascular Emergencies.*) (A), (B), (C), male sex, diabetes, family history of premature heart disease or stroke, obesity, and lack of exercise are all risk factors. (D) is incorrect because a family history of peptic ulcer disease is unrelated to coronary artery disease.

366. **The answer is C.** (Caroline/Little Brown, *Cardiovascular Emergencies.*) (C) is the correct description of the pathophysiology of angina pectoris. (A), (B), and (D) are incorrect.

367. **The answer is A.** (Brady, *Cardiovascular Emergencies.*) (A) is correct and may be accompanied by T-wave inversions. (B), (C), and (D) are incorrect.

368. **The answer is B.** (Brady, *Cardiovascular Emergencies.*) (B) is the correct answer. Most treatment protocols are directed toward the patient with ischemic chest pain, whether due to angina pectoris or an acute myocardial infarction. (A), (C), and (D) are incorrect.

369. **The answer is C.** (Caroline/Little Brown, *Cardiovascular Emergencies.*) (A), (B), (D), putting the patient at ease, putting the patient on a stretcher to rest, beginning an IV, and recording vital signs are the first priorities. (C) is incorrect because, after the first treatment priorities are completed, a 12-lead ECG can be performed.

370. **The answer is B.** (Mosby, *Cardiovascular Emergencies.*) (A), (C), (D), heart failure/pulmonary edema, syncope, and nonlethal dysrhythmias are some of the complications of an acute myocardial infarction. (B) is incorrect because brain tumors are unrelated to an acute myocardial infarction.

371. The answer is D. (Caroline/Little Brown, *Cardiovascular Emergencies.*) (A), (B), and (C) are correct. (D) is incorrect because 10 to 20 percent of acute myocardial infarction patients do not have chest pain and are referred to as silent myocardial infarctions.

372. The answer is D. (Brady, *Cardiovascular Emergencies.*) (A); (B); (C); slow, normal, or fast heart rate; regular or irregular pulse rate; and weak or bounding pulse are all hemodynamic states in an acute myocardial infarction. (D) is incorrect because, even though a normal or increased respiratory rate may be associated with an acute myocardial infarction, it is not a hemodynamic parameter.

373. The answer is C. (Brady, *Cardiovascular Emergencies.*) (A) is important for detecting dysrhythmias, (B) for detecting hemodynamic changes, and (D) for any evidence of left-sided heart failure. (C) is a useful sign for detecting dehydration but is not a significant parameter to be followed in an acute MI patient.

374. The answer is C. (Caroline/Little Brown, *Cardiovascular Emergencies.*) (C) is correct because inverted P waves are not related to an acute myocardial infarction. ST-segment depression and T-wave inversion may be early signs of an acute myocardial infarction or just myocardial ischemia. ST-segment elevation is almost always due to acute myocardial injury from an acute myocardial infarction, but, rarely, coronary artery vasospasm may produce this change as well. (A), (B), (D), tall peaked T waves, and Q waves may all be evolutionary ECG changes seen in an acute myocardial infarction.

375. The answer is A. (Caroline/Little Brown, *Cardiovascular Emergencies.*) (B), (C), (D), systolic blood pressure above 80 and below 180 mmHg, diastolic blood pressure below 120 mmHg, and the patient's being alert and able to give informed consent are all inclusion criteria for thrombolytic therapy. (A) is incorrect because age over 30 years is the correct inclusion criterion.

376. The answer is C. (Caroline/Little Brown, *Cardiovascular Emergencies.*) (C) is correct because, with the bleeding from his right ankle, he is excluded. Other exclusion criteria are oral anticoagulants, major surgery, recent CPR, severe high blood pressure, terminal illness, insulin-dependent diabetes, bleeding disorder, gastrointestinal or genitourinary bleeding, and stroke or transient ischemic attack. (A), (B), and (D) are incorrect because this patient shows no evidence of having these exclusion criteria.

377. Answers.
   (A) 3
   (B) 6
   (C) 4
   (D) 7
   (E) 5
   (F) 2
   (G) 8
   (H) 1

378. Answers.

    (A) 5

    (B) 3

    (C) 1

    (D) 4

    (E) 2

379. The answer is D. (Caroline/Little Brown, *Cardiovascular Emergencies.*) (A), (B), (C), dysrhythmias, and various myocardial muscle diseases (cardiomyopathies) are all causes of left ventricular congestive heart failure. (D) is incorrect because advanced COPD eventually may result in pulmonary artery hypertension, which may result in right, not left, ventricular heart failure.

380. The answer is D. (Caroline/Little Brown, *Cardiovascular Emergencies.*) (A), (B), (C), confusion, agitation, and diaphoresis are all symptoms of left ventricular heart failure. (D) is incorrect because headache is not related to left ventricular heart failure.

381. The answer is B. (Brady, *Cardiovascular Emergencies.*) (A), (C), and (D) are all signs of acute pulmonary edema due to acute left ventricular heart failure. (B) is incorrect because absent pulses are not considered a sign of acute pulmonary edema.

382. The answer is B. (Brady, *Cardiovascular Emergencies.*) (A), (C), and (D) are possible causes of precipitating pulmonary edema. (B) is incorrect because strep throat will not precipitate acute pulmonary edema.

383. The answer is C. (Caroline/Little Brown, *Cardiovascular Emergencies.*) (A), (B), and (D) are all a part of the emergent treatment of a patient with acute pulmonary edema. (C) is a correct drug for the treatment of acute pulmonary edema as well; however, the dosage is usually 20 to 40 mg, not 5 mg, IV bolus.

384. The answer is D. (Brady, *Cardiovascular Emergencies.*) (D) is correct because morphine results in less blood returning to the fluid-overloaded failing heart. (A), (B), and (C) are also actions of morphine but are not of prime importance.

385. The answer is D. (Caroline/Little Brown, *Chest Injuries.*) (D) is the correct definition of cardiac tamponade. (A) and (B) are incorrect because, with cardiac tamponade, as blood fills the pericardium, the coronary arteries and aortic and mitral valves are usually not directly affected. (C) is incorrect because, with cardiac tamponade, the blood pressure usually decreases dramatically.

386. The answer is C. (Caroline/Little Brown, *Chest Injuries.*) (A), (B), (D), narrowed pulse pressure, pulsus paradoxicus, and pale, cool, clammy skin are all clinical signs of cardiac tamponade. (C) is incorrect because one of the classic signs of cardiac tamponade is the presence of "muffled" heart sounds, not clear crisp heart sounds.

387. The answer is A. (Caroline/Little Brown, *Cardiovascular Emergencies*.) (A) is the correct answer because cancer is unrelated to hypertension. (B), (C), and (D) are all examples of end-organ damage, which may be part of the presentation of a hypertensive emergency.

388. The answer is A. (Mosby/ACEP, *Cardiovascular Conditions*.) (B), (C), and (D) are all treatment options available for the prehospital treatment of a hypertensive emergency. (A) is incorrect because dilantin is not a part of the treatment of hypertensive emergencies, but is frequently used for treatment of status epilepticus.

389. The answer is C. (Mosby, *Cardiovascular Emergencies*.) (A), (B), (D), pulmonary congestion, hypoxemia, acidosis, and altered mental status are all signs of cardiogenic shock. (C) is incorrect because marked hypotension, not hypertension, is a sign of cardiogenic shock.

390. The answer is D. (Caroline/Little Brown, *Cardiovascular Emergencies*.) (D) is correct. Most prehospital protocols recommend dopamine over norepinephrine and other vasopressors because its initial doses maintain renal perfusion, unlike most other agents. (A) is incorrect because, even though it is an agent frequently used for cardiogenic shock patients, it is not felt to be the best initial option. (B) is a medication frequently used for treating patients with congestive heart failure but does not have a role in the treatment of cardiogenic shock. (C) is incorrect because the use of MAST trousers in cardiogenic shock is truly controversial and is contraindicated if the patient also has acute pulmonary edema.

391. The answer is B. (Mosby/ACEP, *The Patient without a Pulse*.) (A), (C), (D), major trauma, angina, dysrhythmias, and electrocution are some of the emergent conditions that may progress to cardiac arrest. (B) is incorrect because the viral flu syndrome does not usually progress to cardiac arrest.

392. The answer is A. (Mosby/ACEP, *The Patient without a Pulse*.) (B), (C), (D), and ventricular tachycardia without a pulse are the most common conditions associated with the cardiac arrest patient. (A) is associated with taking digoxin and sometimes with an acute myocardial infarction.

393. The answer is D. (Mosby/ACEP, *The Patient without a Pulse*.) (D) is correct because, in the cardiac arrest patient, you immediately need to know the type of cardiac rhythm, so that you can institute the correct cardiac arrest treatment protocol. (A) is incorrect, because the patient is apneic and would not benefit at all from an oxygen mask, nor from (B) because assessing the need for defibrillation is the first priority. (C) is incorrect, because nitroglycerin is indicated in chest pain patients and acute pulmonary edema patients, but is of no benefit in the cardiac arrest patient.

394. The answer is A. (Brady, *Cardiovascular Emergencies*.) (B), (C), (D), hypoxia, hypothermia, massive pulmonary embolism, drug overdose, hyperkalemia, acidosis, and massive myocardial infarction are all potentially correctable causes of PEA. (A) is incorrect because hyperventilation is a benign, anxiety-related condition, unrelated to cardiac arrest and PEA.

395. Answers. (Brady, *Cardiovascular Emergencies.*)
(A) 3 or 5
(B) 2
(C) 6
(D) 4
(E) 1
(F) 3 or 5

396. The answer is A. (Mosby, *Cardiovascular Emergencies.*) (B), (C), (D), and starting CPR are all critical actions in caring for the cardiac arrest patient. (A) is incorrect because IV calcium is no longer considered useful in the management of the cardiac arrest patient in most cardiac arrest prehospital protocols. However, the use of IV calcium is believed to still be indicated in the cardiac arrest patient with hypocalcemia or with a calcium-blocker medication overdose.

397. The answer is D. (Caroline/Little Brown, *Cardiovascular Emergencies.*) (A), (B), and (C) are accepted criteria for terminating resuscitative efforts. However, it is very important for you to be aware of your state and local laws as well as medical direction guidelines pertaining to this topic.

398. The answer is C. (Brady, *Cardiovascular Emergencies.*) (C) is correct. (A) is incorrect because acute phlebitis, also known as deep-vein thrombosis, usually presents as a hot, red, swollen leg with good motion and normal arterial pulses. (B) is incorrect because it usually presents similarly to phlebitis. (D) is incorrect because acute arthritis presents with a hot, swollen, tender joint.

399. The answer is B. (Brady, *Cardiovascular Emergencies.*) (B) is correct. While this patient may have presented with any of the four rhythms, atrial fibrillation is the only rhythm that is known, over time, to produce thrombus in the atria, which could embolize to an extremity or the brain, resulting in an acute arterial occlusion. (A), (C), and (D) are incorrect because they are not causes of arterial occlusion.

400. The answer is D. (Mosby/ACEP, *Condition by Diagnosis.*) (D) is correct and usually occurs in an artery. (A) is incorrect because the aneurysm may or may not result in a blocking of a vessel. (B) is incorrect because, even though it may be pulsating, it may or may not result in narrowing of a vessel. (C) is incorrect because, even though it may be congenital, it affects the wall of any vessel, not just a vein.

401. **The answer is C.** (Mosby/ACEP, *Condition by Diagnosis.*) (C) is correct and is usually intermittent, associated with walking a certain distance and relieved with rest. It is caused by atherosclerosis and results in arterial narrowing to a leg. (A), (B), and (D) are incorrect.

402. **The answer is D.** (Brady, *Cardiovascular Emergencies.*) (A), (B), (C), infectious, and dissecting are types of aneurysms. (D) is incorrect because sometimes aneurysms may produce thrombus, which may on occasion embolize downstream to an artery, but this is not a type of aneurysm.

403. **The answer is A.** (Mosby/ACEP, *Conditions by Diagnosis.*) (A) is correct because of the ripping quality and the migratory location of the chest pain, but also because of the inequality of the arterial pulses and/or blood pressures in the upper extremities. As the thoracic aorta dissects, the opening to the aortic branches may be sheared off or significantly narrowed, resulting in a significant reduction in arterial blood flow to that affected artery. (B) is incorrect because, although the patient had substernal chest pain, it is usually not ripping in quality and usually does not migrate to another area, and usually any effect on the circulation is symmetrical. (C) is incorrect because an arterial occlusion is usually not associated with chest pain. (D) is incorrect because peptic ulcer disease is not associated with unequal blood pressures, even though chest pain moving to the epigastric area could be suggestive of an ulcer.

404. **The answer is D.** (Mosby/ACEP, *Conditions by Diagnosis.*) (D) is correct. (A) is incorrect because, while the patient may have severe acute abdominal pain, it is usually not with severe hypotension and never with a pulsatile mass. (B) is incorrect because low back strain is never associated with severe hypotension and a pulsatile abdominal mass. (C) is incorrect because, while the patient may have abdominal pain and a large abdominal mass, which is a distended urinary bladder, it is not pulsatile and is not associated with hypotension.

405. **The answer is D.** (Mosby/ACEP, *Conditions by Diagnosis.*) (A), (B), (C), and rapid transport are parts of the emergent care of a patient with an abdominal aortic aneurysm. (D) is incorrect because the hypotensive patient may actually have a leaking or a contained rupture of the abdominal aortic aneurysm, and rapid transport is the first priority. The aneurysm needs to be immediately surgically repaired before it fully ruptures, which may result in hemorrhagic shock and/or cardiac arrest.

406. **The answer is B.** (Brady, *Cardiovascular Emergencies.*) (A), (C), (D), obesity, and lack of exercise are all modifiable risk factors for cardiovascular disease. (B), sex, advanced age, and diabetes are nonmodifiable risk factors. However, there is an opinion that good control of diabetes may reduce the risk as well.

MEDICAL NEUROLOGY

Directions: Each item below contains four suggested responses. Select the **one best** response to each item.

407. Neurological emergencies are often a consequence of all of the following EXCEPT

(A) circulatory changes
(B) intracranial pressure changes
(C) head trauma
(D) intravascular protein concentration changes

408. The main reason an increase in intracranial volume results in a significant increase in intracranial pressure is

(A) the change in brain oncotic pressure
(B) because the skull is a rigid, closed space
(C) the cerebral collateral blood supply
(D) the volume of cerebrospinal fluid

409. After evaluating a patient with any type of nontraumatic neurological emergency, the primary survey includes all of the following EXCEPT

(A) establish and maintain the airway
(B) circulation: check for a pulse
(C) breathing: make sure depth and rate are adequate
(D) drawing baseline blood work

410. All of the following are examples of patients with altered mental status EXCEPT

(A) speaking in a foreign language
(B) syncope
(C) seizures
(D) coma

411. All of the following are possible causes of coma EXCEPT

(A) antibiotics
(B) alcohol
(C) drug overdose
(D) hypoglycemia

412. You are dispatched to the home of a 46-year-old male who is unresponsive. As you arrive in the patient's bedroom, the patient's wife states that he failed to awaken in the morning and she thought that he was sleeping late. However, after 2 hours, she decided to awaken him but was unable to do so. She states that he was known to have hypertension and that he drank socially but went to bed normally last night. The patient's wife denies all questions related to other possible causes of coma. As you begin to examine the patient, you begin by establishing an airway, initiating breathing without a problem, and noting that the patient's pulse and blood pressure are normal. All of the following are important next steps in examining the comatose patient EXCEPT

(A) Check the response to pain.
(B) Check pupillary response.
(C) Check for any nasal discharge.
(D) Check for eye response.

413. You are dispatched to a business office for an unconscious 52-year-old male. This patient delivers supplies to this company, but no one is aware of his medical history. A search of his wallet and clothing fails to reveal any additional information. The patient's assessment reveals stable vital signs and that he is not responsive to any stimuli. After cervical spine immobilization, securing a stable airway, and confirming adequate breathing and circulation, all of the following are parts of the emergent management of this patient EXCEPT

(A) Perform a finger-stick glucose test or draw a blood glucose sample, and then administer 50 mL (25 g) of 50 percent dextrose IV push and repeat as necessary.
(B) If a narcotic overdose is suspected, administer 1 to 2 mg IV, endotracheally, intramuscularly, or SC, and repeat at 2- to 3-minute intervals.
(C) If the patient is an alcoholic, administer 100 mg of thiamine.
(D) If increased intracranial pressure is suspected, hypoventilate the patient at 10 breaths per minute.

414. Which of the following is the correct definition of *seizure*?

(A) A permanent alteration in behavior due to an electrical discharge of a neuron or group of neurons.
(B) A complete loss of consciousness due to a cardiac dysrhythmia.
(C) A temporary alteration of behavior due to an electrical discharge of a neuron or group of neurons.
(D) A temporary alteration of behavior due to a cardiac dysrhythmia.

415. Which of the following is considered the most common cause of seizures?

(A) brain tumor
(B) epileptic patient's failure to take prescribed medications
(C) meningitis
(D) head trauma

416. All of the following are known types of seizures EXCEPT

(A) petit mal seizures
(B) grand mal seizures
(C) allergic seizures
(D) psychomotor seizures

417. Your ambulance is flagged down outside a bar, and a customer states that the patient appeared to have a seizure. The patient had been drinking all afternoon and had stated that he was having problems at home and at work. As a result, the patient stated that he was binge drinking and not taking his medications. The patient was noted to fall abruptly to the floor and began to have dramatic movements of all four extremities. A physical examination revealed that the patient had become incontinent of urine and was now unconscious yet had an adequate airway, was breathing adequately, and had a strong pulse with a blood pressure of 112/76. All of the following are additional priorities for the physical examination of this patient EXCEPT

(A) Examine for any evidence of head trauma.
(B) Examine for pupillary size and reaction to light.
(C) Examine for leg swelling.
(D) Examine for any signs of additional trauma secondary to the seizure activity.

418. All of the following are phases of a generalized, grand mal seizure EXCEPT

(A) aura
(B) hypotonic phase
(C) clonic phase
(D) postictal phase

419. You are dispatched to the scene of a seizing patient. As you arrive at an office building, another employee states that this patient has had a long history of seizures. Today, he was found on the floor of his office actively seizing. The patient was noted to have tonic-clonic contractions of his arms and legs for about 10 minutes, which stopped about 2 minutes ago. As you begin to examine the patient, you note that he is unresponsive and yet his airway appears open and he does not accept an oropharyngeal airway. While placing the patient on a stretcher, he begins again to have another generalized seizure. Treatment of this seizure may include all of the following EXCEPT

(A) Continue to open and maintain the airway.
(B) Administer IV 100 mg of thiamine.
(C) Administer IV 100 g of 50 percent dextrose.
(D) Administer IV slowly up to 10 mg of diazepam (Valium).

420. You are dispatched to a bingo game where an 80-year-old female has passed out. As you arrive at the patient's side, a neighbor states that she had become very excited and admitted to feeling a little dizzy because she had just won the grand prize. Upon yelling out "bingo" and jumping up, she passed out and landed on the floor. After about a minute, she woke up. As you begin to obtain a history from the patient, she notes that she has just had a yearly physical examination and has not had any significant medical problems. She had her appendix out 40 years ago and a hysterectomy 30 years ago. She does not take any medications. She does admit to passing out several years ago at a funeral and having a similar light-headed feeling before passing out. You next begin to examine the patient in order to determine the cause of the syncopal episode. All of the following areas of physical examination would help to determine the cause of the syncope EXCEPT

(A) searching for a skin rash
(B) pulse rate
(C) blood pressure, supine and erect
(D) focal weakness

421. Match the following symptoms or physical findings with the list of causes of syncope.

(A) postural increase in pulse rate of 20 beats per minute, decrease in systolic blood pressure of 20 mmHg
(B) pulse 30 beats per minute, blood pressure 50 palpable
(C) pulse 180 beats per minute, blood pressure 62/46
(D) finger-stick glucose level 42
(E) unconsciousness, urinary incontinence, and confusion upon awakening

1. Stokes-Adams syncope due to tachy- or bradydysrhythmia
2. seizure disorder
3. acute gastrointestinal bleeding
4. vasovagal syncope
5. hypoglycemia

422. As you await the end of a busy day, you are dispatched to a 74-year-old male who has just "passed out" at home. Upon your arrival, you find the patient lying on the floor. He apologizes for his wife's calling the ambulance because he truly feels fine now. The patient's wife interrupts by stating that he was simply walking across the room and suddenly fainted and hit the floor without any warning. His wife stated that he was unconscious for about 2 minutes but then awakened without any signs of confusion, weakness, slurred speech, or headache. As you examine the patient, you note that he has normal vital signs without orthostatic changes, and an initial survey reveals only abrasions of both knees. The patient also is alert; oriented to person, place, and time; and has grossly symmetrical neurological findings. The appropriate prehospital management of this patient includes all of the following EXCEPT

(A) encouraging the patient to be released against medical advice
(B) high-flow oxygen
(C) IV to keep vein open
(D) cardiac monitoring

423. You are dispatched to a patient with a severe headache who is frightened. As you arrive at the patient's home, you find a 42-year-old male who is grimacing with his head in his hands, stating that about 25 minutes ago, he experienced the worst headache in his life. He noted that his day began as usual, with breakfast and dressing to go to work, when he experienced an acute left-sided headache. Upon further questioning, he admitted to rarely having mild to moderate headaches, one to two times a year, which immediately resolved with aspirin or Tylenol. Today, the headache was so intense that the Tylenol did nothing, and the severity of the headache persisted. Your initial physical examination reveals that the patient is afebrile to touch and has a blood pressure of 124/78, a regular pulse of 88 beats per minute, respirations of 20 breaths per minute, pupils that are equal and reactive to light, and normal gross neurological findings. All of the following are signs or symptoms that would heighten your concerns of a possibly serious or potentially life-threatening cause of a headache EXCEPT

(A) Patient complains of a fever and a stiff neck.
(B) Patient complains of congestion, with facial and forehead pain and tenderness.
(C) Patient demonstrates focal neurologic abnormality.
(D) Patient has a bleeding disorder or is taking blood-thinning medication.

424. Match the following types of headache with the appropriate pathophysiologic or identifying characteristic.

(A) tension
(B) sinus
(C) migraine
(D) meningitis
(E) hypertensive
(F) subarachnoid hemorrhage
(G) toxic exposure

1. throbbing headache, often with nausea and vomiting
2. fever and stiff neck
3. stress-related, in the front of the head to the occipital area
4. sudden onset of worse headache, vomiting, and stiff neck
5. associated with confusion, chest tightness, and fumes
6. associated with diastolic blood pressure above 120 mmHg
7. nasal congestion, forehead or cheek tenderness

425. Which of the following is the most accurate description of the most likely clinical presentation of a patient with a brain tumor?

(A) sudden onset of headache associated with coma
(B) fever, chills, and stiff neck
(C) memory difficulty and personality change over a long period of time
(D) head trauma followed by seizures

426. You are stopped at an intersection when a teenage boy runs out in front of the ambulance to ask for your help. His mother was told 6 months ago that she has a malignant brain tumor on the right side of her brain. This morning she had difficulty climbing out of bed and needed assistance because of weakness. As you enter the patient's bedroom, you find the patient lying in bed with a blank stare on her face. As you begin to examine the patient, you find focal weakness. With this presentation, you would expect to find the weakness in which of the following areas?

(A) left upper and/or lower extremity
(B) right upper and/or lower extremity
(C) bilateral upper extremity weakness
(D) bilateral lower extremity weakness

427. All of the following are examples of critical signs of a probable neurological or medical emergency EXCEPT

(A) a single dilated, unreactive pupil
(B) memory deficit
(C) decreasing level of responsiveness
(D) unresponsiveness with elevated blood pressure

428. All of the following are mechanisms of strokes EXCEPT

(A) thrombotic
(B) embolic
(C) metastatic
(D) hemorrhagic

429. A stroke leads to weakness, paralysis, speech disorders, confusion, coma, and other acute neurologic deficits that are due to which of the following?

(A) seizure

(B) acute increase in intracranial pressure

(C) brain metastasis

(D) sudden vascular catastrophe

430. You are dispatched to a nursing home for a 78-year-old male with an acute onset of confusion and left-sided weakness. The nurse on the floor notes that the patient has a history of hypertension and an old left-sided cerebrovascular accident, resulting in right-leg weakness. On review of last evening's nurse's notes, it is found that the patient did complain of a mild headache, which responded to two aspirin. At present, the patient is too confused to answer any of your questions concerning this episode. All of the following are physical findings due to an acute stroke EXCEPT

(A) focal hemiparesis or hemiplegia (opposite to the side of the brain damage)

(B) dysarthria

(C) hypertension and bradycardia

(D) leg edema

431. All of the following are correct statements concerning an acute hemorrhagic stroke EXCEPT

(A) The two types are intracerebral hemorrhage and subxyphoid hemorrhage.

(B) The mortality rate is 50 to 80 percent

(C) The average age is fifties to early sixties.

(D) Patients frequently have a history of high blood pressure.

432. You are dispatched to a business office for a 56-year-old female complaining of a severe headache. Upon your arrival, you find the patient lying on a couch in the lobby. The patient notes that she has been under the care of an internist for hypertension, which runs throughout her entire family. Today, she awoke and went to work and felt normal. Then, about an hour ago, she felt an acute onset of the worst headache of her entire life. She also notes that she feels pain in her neck and then down her back, associated with feeling very nauseous. As you begin to assess the patient and your partner begins to take the patient's vital signs, you note that the patient is acting confused and becoming more somnolent. Since the only abnormality on physical examination is elevated blood pressure of 178/124 bilaterally and the patient has grossly symmetrical neurological findings, you suspect that the cause of the patient's symptoms is which of the following events?

(A) acute meningitis

(B) brain tumor

(C) thrombosed cerebral vessel

(D) ruptured cerebral aneurysm

433. You are called to respond to a possible stroke patient. When you arrive at the patient's apartment, you find an 86-year-old male who awoke feeling weak. Upon arising to get out of bed, the patient noted that his right leg was dragging, and his friend could not understand him on the telephone. Upon examining the patient, you note that his blood pressure is 186/120 bilaterally, his speech is truly slurred, and he has 2 out of 4 strength in his right arm and 1 out of 4 strength in his right leg. All of the following are appropriate treatment options for this patient EXCEPT

(A) Establish and maintain the airway.
(B) Administer oxygen and attach the patient to an ECG monitor.
(C) Request permission to open and administer a sublingual nifedipine capsule to lower the blood pressure.
(D) Protect the paretic limbs in order to prevent injury during transport.

434. As you proceed to an 88-year-old female with a stroke at the Sunshine Nursing Home, you jest with your partner as to what the true nature of this call could be. Yet, as you arrive at the patient's bedside, you note that several members of the staff are very upset with the patient's condition. Evidently, the patient awoke complaining of a headache and then gradually became more confused, with left-sided upper and lower extremity paralysis. After the staff called 911, the patient became barely responsive to verbal stimuli and responsive to painful stimuli. Your assessment of this very lethargic patient revealed that she had a blood pressure of 168/104 bilaterally, symmetrical pupils that reacted to light, an absent gag reflex, and insignificant findings on the remainder of the physical examination. However, the patient's neurological examination documented that the patient had left-sided flaccid paralysis. All of the following are parts of the emergency care rendered to this patient EXCEPT

(A) Perform a finger-stick glucose determination, and treat hypoglycemia if present.
(B) Immediately perform endotracheal intubation.
(C) Hyperventilate the patient.
(D) Transport in the stable side position.

435. Transient ischemic attacks are episodes of focal neurologic deficits, similar to cerebrovascular accidents, that totally resolve within

(A) 1 hour
(B) 8 to10 hours
(C) 24 hours
(D) 24 to 48 hours

436. A transient ischemic attack is clinically most important because it is a reliable sign of an impending

(A) sudden death
(B) stroke
(C) acute myocardial infarction
(D) status epilepticus

437. You arrive at a senior-citizen center to find a 75-year-old male who complains that, at lunch about an hour ago, he noticed that his left hand became numb and weak and he spilled his coffee. He is embarrassed because the supervisor of the center called for the ambulance. He notes that his hand has come back to normal in the past 5 minutes, and he desires to simply go home. Upon your examination, the patient has a blood pressure of 156/102, a regular pulse of 86 beats per minute, and respiration at 18 breaths per minute. His physical examination findings are grossly normal, and his neurologic assessment reveals symmetrical motor and sensory findings, with orientation to person, place, and time. While the patient is playing down his complaints and wants to sign out against medical advice, you and the center's supervisor are successful in convincing the patient to go to the hospital. During transport, the patient again notes that he is feeling numbness and weakness in his left hand. Your assessment confirms that the patient's strength in the hand is 2 out of 4, and his blood pressure is now 156/100 bilaterally. All of the following are part of the emergency care rendered to this patient EXCEPT

(A) Establish and maintain the airway.
(B) Administer oxygen.
(C) Administer sublingual nifedipine to lower the blood pressure.
(D) Start an IV with normal saline solution or lactated Ringer's solution.

438. All of the following are symptoms or
signs of transient ischemic attacks
EXCEPT

(A) monocular blindness
(B) staggering gait
(C) constipation
(D) numbness and/or paresthesias

MEDICAL
NEUROLOGY

ANSWERS

407. The answer is D. (Mosby, *Nervous System Disorders*.) (D) is correct because changes in the intravascular protein concentration can effect the overall health of all patients but are not often causes of neurologic emergencies. (A) Circulatory changes such as acute cerebrovascular accident or shock of multiple etiologies are examples of neurologic emergencies. (B) from any traumatic injury to the brain or from a growing brain tumor may increase intracranial pressure and produce a neurologic emergency. (C), in the form of a penetrating or nonpenetrating trauma, is an example of a neurologic emergency.

408. The answer is B. (Mosby, *Nervous System Disorders*.) (B) is the reason that any increase in intracranial volume results in a significant increase in intracranial pressure. (A), (C), and (D) are incorrect.

409. The answer is D. (Caroline/Little Brown, *Unconscious States*.) (A), (B), and (C) are parts of the primary survey and are the first priority for the treatment of nontraumatic neurologic emergencies. (D) is incorrect because baseline blood work will be helpful but is of little use in the prehospital setting and certainly is not as important as the airway, breathing, and circulation.

410. The answer is A. (Mosby/ACEP, *Altered Mental Status*.) (B), (C), (D), disorientation, and strange behavior are all examples of patients presenting with an altered mental status. (A) is not an example of a patient with an altered mental status.

411. The answer is A. (Caroline/Little Brown, *Unconscious States*.) (B), (C), and (D) are all part of the pneumonic AEIOU TIPS, which outlines some of the most common causes of coma: A = alcohol or acidosis; E = epilepsy, electrolyte abnormality, or endocrine problem; I = insulin (hypoglycemia); O = overdose; U = uremia; T = trauma or temperature abnormality; I = infection (meningitis); P = psychogenic; S = stroke or space-occupying cerebral lesion. (A) is incorrect because, while antibiotics might produce certain side effects and toxic effects, they are not associated with causing coma.

412. **The answer is C.** (Brady, *Nervous System Emergencies*.) (A) is important in determining any focal abnormality. (B) is important, since unilateral dilation of a pupil implies pressure on the third cranial nerve, while bilateral mid-sized pupils are suggestive of a midbrain lesion, and pinpoint pupils may be caused by a lesion in the pons. (D) is important because dysconjugate gaze (eyes looking in different directions) at rest implies a structural brain-stem injury. (C) is incorrect because, other than looking for the presence of blood or cerebrospinal fluid in nasal discharge in the head trauma patient, the evaluation of nasal discharge is not important in the comatose patient.

413. **The answer is D.** (Brady, *Nervous System Emergencies*.) (A), (B), and (C) are parts of the emergent management of the patient with an altered mental status. (D) is incorrect because, if increased intracranial pressure is suspected, hyperventilation will result in lowering the carbon dioxide level in the blood, which will result in cerebral vasoconstriction and will minimize brain swelling.

414. **The answer is C.** (Brady, *Nervous System Emergencies*; Mosby, *Nervous System Disorders*.) (C) is the correct definition. (A) is incorrect because a seizure is temporary, not permanent. (B) is incorrect because this is the definition of Stokes-Adam syncope. (D) is incorrect because the definition of seizure is unrelated to a cardiac dysrhythmia.

415. **The answer is B.** (Caroline/Little Brown, *Unconscious States*.) (B) is correct because it is accepted as the most common cause of seizures. (A), (C), (D), hypoxia, hypoglycemia, toxins, drugs, drug withdrawal, eclampsia of pregnancy, and idiopathic (unknown cause) are all causes of seizures, but not the most common cause.

416. **The answer is C.** (Brady, *Nervous System Emergencies*.) (C) is correct because there is no such entity as an allergic seizure. (A), (B), (D), and focal motor are all types of true seizures. Hysterical seizures are demonstrated by patients with psychological problems.

417. **The answer is C.** (Caroline/Little Brown, *Unconscious States*.) (A); (B); (D); examine the mouth for any evidence of mouth trauma; examine for neck rigidity; examine the extremities for any signs of trauma, medication bracelets, or needle tracks; and examine the patient's clothes and possessions for any evidence of medication vials. (C) is incorrect because leg swelling is usually unrelated to seizures.

418. **The answer is B.** (Brady, *Nervous System Emergencies*.) (A), loss of consciousness, tonic phase, hypertonic phase, (C), postseizure, and (D) are all phases of a generalized, grand mal seizure. (B) is not a phase.

419. The answer is C. (Caroline/Little Brown, *Unconscious States.*) (A), (B), (D), administering high-concentration oxygen, and administering 25 g of 50 percent dextrose are all parts of the treatment of status epilepticus. (C) is incorrect because the correct dosage of 50 percent dextrose is 25 g, not 100 g.

420. The answer is A. (Mosby/ACEP, *Syncope.*) (B) may reveal a dramatically rapid or slow pulse, which may be responsible for syncope. (C) may reveal a 20-mmHg drop in systolic blood pressure, associated with a 20 beat per minute increase in pulse rate, which would be diagnostic of postural hypotension. This is associated with hypovolemia from any possible cause, such as recurrent vomiting or diarrhea, bleeding from any source, or use of diuretics. (D) may be suggestive of a cerebrovascular accident or intracerebral pathology. (A) is incorrect because a skin rash does not provide evidence for a particular cause of syncope.

421. Answers. (Mosby/ACEP, *Syncope*; Caroline/Little Brown, *Unconscious States.*)
  (A) 3
  (B) 4
  (C) 1
  (D) 5
  (E) 2

While 3 could also be the answer for (C), 1 could not be the answer for (A).

422. The answer is A. (Mosby/ACEP, *Syncope.*) (B), (C), (D), transporting the patient in the position of comfort, and treating any specific causes of syncope as well, for example, IV 50 percent dextrose for hypoglycemia. (A) is incorrect because a patient with syncope should be transported to the emergency department in order to determine whether the cause is benign or of a serious nature.

423. The answer is B. (Mosby/ACEP, *Headache.*) (A) is suggestive of possible meningitis (infection of the spinal fluid) until proven otherwise. (C) is strongly suggestive of a structural lesion in the brain, such as a cerebrovascular accident, intracerebral hemorrhage, subdural or epidural hematoma, and so on. (D) is always worrisome because one of the potentially most serious clinical presentations in such patients is an acute intracerebral hemorrhage, resulting in a critical neurologic injury. (B) is incorrect because these symptoms are suggestive of acute sinusitis that is usually not serious or life threatening.

424. Answers. (Mosby/ACEP, *Headache.*)
  (A) 3
  (B) 7
  (C) 1
  (D) 2
  (E) 6
  (F) 4
  (G) 5

425. **The answer is C.** (Mosby/ACEP, *Altered Mental Status.*) (C) is correct, and these changes may also be associated with a recurrent headache. (A) is often the presentation of an intracerebral or subarachnoid hemorrhage. (B) is suspicious for meningitis. (D) is a complication of head trauma and unrelated to a brain tumor.

426. **The answer is A.** (Mosby/ACEP, *Altered Mental Status.*) (A) is correct, since the malignant tumor lies on the right side of the patient's brain and would be expected to produce left-sided weakness. These findings are the same as for an acute cerebrovascular accident on the right side of the brain. (B), (C), and (D) are incorrect.

427. **The answer is B.** (Mosby/ACEP, *Altered Mental Status.*) (A) is suggestive of increased intracranial pressure and possible irreversible brain damage. (C) is also a sign of an acute medical emergency that may be life-threatening. (D) is usually a sign of intracranial bleeding or swelling. (B) is incorrect because the most common cause of memory deficit is chronic dementia, often from Alzheimer's disease or multiple cerebral infarcts.

428. **The answer is C.** (Caroline/Little Brown, *Unconscious States.*) (A) is responsible for 60 percent of all strokes and is due to atherosclerosis. (B) is known for its abrupt onset. (D) actually is representative of intracerebral hemorrhage and subarachnoid hemorrhage. (C) is incorrect because, while many malignancies metastasize (spread) to the brain, this mechanism has nothing to do with strokes.

429. **The answer is D.** (Caroline/Little Brown, *Unconscious States.*) (D) is the correct explanation for the cause of the stroke. (A), (B), and (C) are all possible causes of neurologic injury but are not known to produce a stroke.

430. **The answer is D.** (Caroline/Little Brown, *Unconscious States.*) (A), (B), (C), seizures, coma, inappropriate affect, expressive and/or receptive aphasia, irregular pulse, staggering gait, and stiff neck are all possible findings due to a stroke. (D) is unrelated to a stroke.

431. **The answer is A.** (Caroline/Little Brown, *Unconscious States*; Mosby, *Nervous System Disorders.*) (B), (C), and (D) are correct. (A) is incorrect because the two types of acute hemorrhagic strokes are intracerebral hemorrhage and subarachnoid hemorrhage. There is no such thing as a subxyphoid hemorrhage.

432. **The answer is D.** (Caroline/Little Brown, *Unconscious States.*) (D) is correct. This presentation is classic for a subarachnoid hemorrhage, which is due to a ruptured cerebral aneurysm. (A) is incorrect because the presentation is usually a gradual onset of fever and progressive generalized illness associated with stiff neck and toxic appearance. (B) is incorrect because a brain tumor usually causes a very slow and gradual deterioration of mental and physical functioning over months. (C) is incorrect because a thrombosed cerebral vessel usually presents with focal neurologic abnormalities and also causes a slowly progressive deterioration of functions, not abrupt changes, as in this patient.

433. The answer is C. (Caroline/Little Brown, *Unconscious States.*) (A), (B), and (D) are correct treatment of the patient with an acute ischemic or hemorrhagic stroke. (C) is incorrect because, in the presence of an acute ischemic stroke, the abrupt lowering of the blood pressure may be dangerous and may actually increase the amount of brain damage.

434. The answer is B. (Brady, *Nervous System Emergencies*; Caroline/Little Brown, *Unconscious States.*) (A) is correct because hypoglycemia may produce an altered mental status sometimes associated with focal neurologic abnormalities. (C) is correct because hyperventilation will produce vasoconstriction of intracerebral blood vessels, which will result in lowering of intracerebral pressure. (D) is correct because the stroke victim, without a gag reflex, is at increased risk of aspiration. Placing the patient on her side will reduce the chance of aspiration. (B) is incorrect because, in the acute stroke victim who is awake, you would try to avoid endotracheal intubation because the attempt may actually cause an increase in intracerebral pressure.

435. The answer is C. (Mosby, *Nervous System Disorders.*) (A) is the correct amount of time within which there is total resolution of symptoms, without any residual neurological deficits.

436. The answer is B. (Mosby, *Nervous System Disorders.*) (B) is correct because, usually within 2 years, a patient with a transient ischemic attack will have an acute stroke. (A), (C), and (D) are all unrelated to the patient experiencing a transient ischemic attack.

437. The answer is C. (Caroline/Little Brown, *Unconscious States.*) (A), (B), (D), assuring patient safety, hyperventilation if the patient is unconscious, drawing a blood sample or finger-stick glucose determination, protecting paralyzed limbs, patient reassurance, and transport without excessive movement are part of the treatment of both a transient ischemic attack and an acute cerebrovascular accident. The treatment is primarily supportive. (C) is incorrect because, in a thrombotic transient ischemic attack or cerebrovascular accident, any decrease in the blood pressure may be dangerous and may actually result in worsening of the deficit.

438. The answer is C. (Brady, *Nervous System Emergencies.*) (A), (B), (D), hemiplegia, hemiparesis, difficulty in swallowing, aphasia, and dizziness are some examples of symptoms or signs of transient ischemic attacks. (C) is incorrect.

ENDOCRINE EMERGENCIES

Directions: Each item below contains four suggested responses. Select the **one best** response to each item.

439. Diabetes mellitus is a disease characterized by a lack of

(A) sodium
(B) potassium
(C) insulin
(D) testosterone

440. Type I diabetes mellitus is characterized by all of the following EXCEPT

(A) inadequate production of insulin
(B) dehydration
(C) accumulation of organic acids and ketones
(D) metabolic alkalosis

441. Which of the following is the correct explanation of the manner in which osmotic diuresis produces dehydration in the type I diabetes mellitus patient?

(A) The elevation of the blood sugar level produces fever, which produces sweating and subsequent dehydration.
(B) As the blood sugar level rises in the blood, it spills into the urine and pulls water with it. This increased urination, known as polyuria, results in dehydration.
(C) Type I diabetes mellitus frequently results in acute kidney damage, which results in dehydration.
(D) As the blood sugar level rises in the urine, this always results in a urinary tract infection, which produces urinary frequency, which results in dehydration.

442. You are dispatched to a "sick" patient and find a 38-year-old male who admits to having diabetes. He complains of having the flu for the past week and has not had much of an appetite. As a result, he has not taken his insulin for 3 days. He now feels very weak and tired and yet has been urinating more than usual. Your assessment reveals a hot-to-touch patient with a blood pressure of 82/52, a pulse of 124 beats per minute, and respirations of 32 breaths per minute, with a patent airway and adequate ventilation. After performing a finger-stick glucose test or obtaining a blood sugar level, the next most important treatment is

(A) 30 units IV NPH insulin
(B) 10 meq potassium chloride
(C) 1 to 2 liters IV 0.9 percent normal saline solution
(D) 1.0 mg IV naloxone (Narcan)

443. You are dispatched to an 18-year-old female who was found unconscious in her college bedroom. Her roommate states that the patient appeared sick and refused to go to the student infirmary. She also states that she has only known the girl for the past 4 weeks but truly believes that the patient showed no signs of alcohol or drug use. Your assessment reveals that this patient is warm to touch and unresponsive to all stimuli. The vital signs are blood pressure of 80 palpable, pulse of 120 beats per minute, and respirations of 22 breaths per minute. As you begin to perform a rapid physical examination, you find a bracelet that states that the patient is a diabetic. Based upon this presentation, after checking the ABCs, the first priority in the management of this patient should consist of which of the following?

(A) immediate administration of 0.9 percent normal saline solution IV
(B) 10 units regular insulin IV
(C) 50 ml 50 percent dextrose
(D) IV epinephrine 1.0 mg of 1:10,000 solution

444. All of the following are correct statements concerning type II diabetes mellitus EXCEPT

(A) It frequently occurs in obese patients.
(B) Obesity causes an increase in blood sugar by converting protein to sugar.
(C) Most patients are treated with diet and oral agents.
(D) It usually occurs in later life, not childhood.

445. All of the following are signs and symptoms of a hypoglycemic reaction EXCEPT

(A) confusion, combative behavior, and irritability

(B) frequent urination, increased thirst, and increased appetite

(C) rapid pulse, and cold and clammy skin

(D) nervousness, drowsiness, and coma

446. All of the following are possible long-term complications of diabetes mellitus EXCEPT

(A) kidney failure

(B) heart disease and strokes

(C) blindness

(D) cirrhosis of the liver

447. You are dispatched to an unresponsive diabetic at work. As you arrive in the factory, you find a 24-year-old male, unresponsive to all stimuli. His co-workers state that the patient was acting strange and arguing vehemently, when he went to the bathroom and did not return for 10 minutes. As his coworkers opened the bathroom door, they found the unresponsive patient lying on the bathroom floor. All of the following are causes of hypoglycemia in diabetic patients EXCEPT

(A) increased intake of carbohydrates in the diet

(B) increased physical activity or exercise

(C) increased insulin or oral hypo-glycemic agents

(D) decreased dietary intake

448. You are dispatched to the home of a 23-year-old female who has been complaining for 2 weeks of gradual weakness associated with increased desire to urinate, drink fluids, and eat. Since she is obese, her family had become suspicious that she had some form of eating disorder and had made an appointment with a special eating center in about 4 weeks. However, in the last 2 days she has simply felt weaker and has been sleeping more, even during most of the day. Finally, she asked for help to go to the bathroom and had to be caught before passing out upon walking. The patient's mother did note that her husband's family had a history of diabetes, with his brother dying at an early age with complications related to it. As you begin to assess this patient, you might expect to find all of the following signs of diabetic ketoacidosis EXCEPT

(A) fruity breath odor

(B) warm, dry skin, with dry parched mucous membranes

(C) hypotension and tachycardia

(D) bradypnea, with a respiratory rate of 6 breaths minute

449. All of the following are symptoms of patients in diabetic ketoacidosis EXCEPT

(A) polyuria, polydypsia, and polyphagia

(B) swollen joints

(C) nausea, vomiting, and severe abdominal pain

(D) weakness, tiredness, and lethargy

450. All of the following are known causes of diabetic ketoacidosis in known diabetics EXCEPT

(A) taking too much insulin
(B) infection
(C) increased stress from surgery or trauma
(D) failing to take insulin

451. All of the following are frequent causes of hypoglycemia in insulin-dependent diabetics EXCEPT

(A) lack of sleep
(B) decreased dietary intake in a patient taking insulin
(C) an error in insulin dosage
(D) a combination of B and C

452. Hypoglycemia is an acute medical emergency because the failure to recognize and correct it may result in which of the following?

(A) permanent brain damage
(B) kidney failure
(C) blindness
(D) acute myocardial infarction

453. You are dispatched to an unconscious male found in an alley. As you arrive at the patient's side, a local bartender identifies the patient as a regular customer at his bar for the past several years. The bartender states that the patient has told him his life's story several times over the years and notes that the patient has high blood pressure and arthritis, and had his appendix removed 2 years ago and fractured his hip 5 years ago. He is adamant that the patient has never had diabetes, nor has anyone in his family. After your partner reveals an overall normal physical and neurological assessment, an argument ensues between the well-meaning bartender and your partner over the need for IV dextrose, since the patient is not a diabetic and has never taken insulin or oral hypoglycemic medications. Acute hypoglycemia may occur in patients with all of the following diseases EXCEPT

(A) certain drug overdoses
(B) certain cancers
(C) alcoholics
(D) prostatism

454. You are completing the assessment and initial management of a 22-year-old homeless diabetic with classic diabetic ketoacidosis and are making final preparations to transport the patient. Suddenly, the Paramedic student riding with you notes that the ECG rhythm strip looks funny. As you and your partner review it, you note that the gross abnormality appears to be very tall, peaked T waves. You quickly change leads and note that it is truly present in each lead checked. In diabetic ketoacidosis, the tall, peaked T waves are due to which of the following abnormalities?

(A) hypernatremia
(B) dehydration
(C) hyperglycemia
(D) hyperkalemia

455. You are called to respond to an emotionally disturbed man. As you pull up to the scene, a police officer tells you to be careful with this emotionally charged patient. A bystander notes that a car was weaving in and out of traffic with an emotionally upset driver. As the police stopped the car, the driver appeared very upset but was making little sense. While you begin to slowly approach the patient, another bystander comes by to tell you that this patient is his neighbor and he believes that he is a diabetic. He recalls a similar episode, when the patient's wife called 911 because he was acting bizarre about 2 years ago. Upon approaching the patient, you note that he is sweating. His vital signs are blood pressure of 126/86, respirations of 18 breaths per minute, and a regular pulse of 156 beats per minute. Your findings upon initial assessment are grossly normal, but you did discover a wrist bracelet that confirms that he is a diabetic on insulin. While the patient will not allow you to perform a finger-stick glucose test or draw blood, he will allow you to treat him to make him feel better. Which of the following is the correct first step in treating this patient?

(A) immediate 50 to 100 ml 50 percent dextrose IV push
(B) nasal oxygen
(C) adenosine 6 mg IV push
(D) oral glucose administration with orange juice, soda, or some form of glucose paste

456. All of the following are correct statements about hyperosmolar hyperglycemic nonketotic coma EXCEPT

   (A) It usually occurs in older patients.
   (B) A 0.9 percent saline solution IV is a priority.
   (C) Ambu-bag hyperventilation is helpful in correcting the keto-acidosis.
   (D) It is sometimes precipitated by certain medications, such as thiazide diuretics or steroids, and sometimes by enteral or parenteral feedings.

457. Hyperthyroidism is a condition consisting of an overactive thyroid gland. All of the following are signs or symptoms of hyperthyroidism EXCEPT

   (A) cold intolerance
   (B) hypertension
   (C) tachycardia
   (D) weight loss

458. All of the following are signs or symptoms of hypothyoidism EXCEPT

   (A) cold intolerance
   (B) lethargy
   (C) altered mental status
   (D) dry skin and brittle hair

459. All of the following are a part of the prehospital emergent treatment of hyper- or hypothyroidism EXCEPT

   (A) ABCs
   (B) cardiac monitoring
   (C) IV digoxin
   (D) IV access

460. Cushing's disease, which is another name for hyperadrenalism, consists of all of the following EXCEPT

   (A) unusual fat distribution
   (B) rapid mood swings
   (C) hyperkalemia
   (D) increased blood sugar

461. Hypoadrenalism, also known as Addison's disease, may present with all of the following signs and symptoms EXCEPT

   (A) hypertension
   (B) nausea and vomiting
   (C) hypoglycemia
   (D) weakness and fatigue

ENDOCRINE EMERGENCIES

ANSWERS

439. The answer is C. (Brady, *Endocrine Emergencies*.) Diabetes mellitus is characterized by decreased secretion of insulin by the pancreas. As a result, blood glucose is unable to enter the cells of the body and builds up in the blood.

440. The answer is D. (Brady, *Endocrine Emergencies*.) (A), (B), and (C) are all characteristics of type I diabetes mellitus. (D) is incorrect because, in type I diabetes mellitus, with the accumulation of organic acids, the patient often develops a metabolic acidosis, not a metabolic alkalosis.

441. The answer is B. (Brady, *Endocrine Emergencies*.) (B) is the manner in which dehydration develops in the type I diabetic patient. (A) is incorrect because an elevated blood sugar level does not produce fever. (C) is incorrect because diabetes does not produce acute kidney damage. Any kidney damage that may occur is a slow, chronic process. (D) is incorrect because an elevated blood sugar level does not always produce a urinary tract infection. Even if a urinary tract infection develops, urinary frequency does not cause dehydration.

442. The answer is C. (Brady, *Endocrine and Metabolic Emergencies*; Mosby/ACEP, *Diabetic Emergencies*.) (C) is correct because the patient has not been taking his insulin and is dehydrated and hypotensive. After ensuring the airway and breathing and assessing the circulation, the first priority is to provide IV fluid replacement for the dehydrated patient. (A) is incorrect because routine administration of intravenous insulin is not a part of prehospital protocols. However, if there was some reason for a delay in transport, medical control may give you permission to help administer the patient's own insulin. Nevertheless, the dose would never be as much as 30 units IV. Finally, in the acute treatment of uncontrolled diabetes, regular (short-acting) insulin is used, not NPH (long-acting) insulin. (B) and (D) have no place in the initial treatment of an acute diabetic emergency.

443. The answer is C. (Mosby/ACEP, *Diabetic Emergencies.*) (C) is correct because all diabetic patients with severely altered mental status need to have IV glucose administration because of the possibility of hypoglycemia causing an altered mental status. (A) is incorrect because IV glucose is the first priority; then IV 0.9 percent normal saline solution may be administered. (B) and (D) are not appropriate.

444. The answer is B. (Brady, *Endocrine Emergencies.*) (A), (C), and (D) are all correct. (B) is incorrect because the increased blood sugar levels in type II diabetes mellitus usually occur when obesity causes a decrease in the number of insulin receptors, which become defective and less responsive to insulin.

445. The answer is B. (Mosby, *Diabetic Emergencies.*) (A), (C), and (D) are correct. (B) is incorrect because these are classic symptoms for hyperglycemia (elevated blood sugar) due to diabetes and are unrelated to hypoglycemia.

446. The answer is D. (Mosby, *Diabetic Emergencies.*) (A), (B), (C), peripheral neuropathy, and autonomic neuropathy are some of the potential long-term complications of diabetes mellitus. (D) is incorrect because it is unrelated to diabetes and is frequently related to alcoholism or chronic hepatitis.

447. The answer is A. (Mosby, *Diabetic Emergencies.*) (B), (C), and (D) are correct. (A) is incorrect because an increased intake of carbohydrates usually results in an increase in blood sugar (hyperglycemia) rather than a decrease (hypoglycemia).

448. The answer is D. (Caroline/Little Brown, *Unconscious States.*) (A), (B), (C), and sometimes fever are common signs of diabetic ketoacidosis. (D) is incorrect because classically, in diabetic ketoacidosis, a lack of insulin produces a very high level of blood sugar, which cannot be utilized by the cells of the body for energy. As a result, the body attempts to compensate by breaking down fats, which generates a large amount of acids and ketones. This results in a severe metabolic acidosis, which the body attempts to compensate for by increasing the respiratory rate and the depth of respirations. This physical finding is known as Kussmaul's respirations and is the body's attempt to blow off carbon dioxide in order to correct the severe metabolic acidosis.

449. The answer is B. (Caroline/Little Brown, *Unconscious States.*) (A), (C), and (D) are common symptoms of patients in diabetic ketoacidosis. Sometimes the severity of the abdominal pain is mistaken for an acute abdomen, and the patient is considered for an acute laparotomy. As the diabetic ketoacidosis is corrected, the nausea, vomiting, and abdominal pain gradually subside. (B) is incorrect because swollen joints are not usually associated with diabetic ketoacidosis but are more frequently seen with various diseases that cause acute arthritis.

450. The answer is A. (Mosby, *Diabetic Emergencies.*) (B), (C), (D), increased dietary intake, and decreased metabolic rate are some of the most common reasons for diabetics to develop diabetic ketoacidosis. Less common causes are pregnancy, increased alcohol intake, and severe emotional stress. (A) is incorrect because increased insulin dose usually results in hypoglycemia, not an elevation of blood sugar with ketoacidosis.

451. **The answer is A.** (Mosby/ACEP, *Diabetic Emergencies.*) (B), (C), and (D) are common causes of hypoglycemia in insulin-dependent diabetics. (A) is incorrect because it is usually not related to hypoglycemia.

452. **The answer is A.** (Brady, *Endocrine and Metabolic Emergencies.*) (A) is correct, primarily because the brain depends on glucose for most of its energy. (B), (C), and (D) are incorrect; they are potential long-term complications of diabetes mellitus and are unrelated to hypoglycemia.

453. **The answer is D.** (Caroline/Little Brown, *Unconscious States.*) (A), (B), (C), liver disease, kidney disease, and certain poisonings may also cause hypoglycemic reactions. You must be very careful to note that a lack of a history of diabetes in an unresponsive patient does not eliminate the possibility of hypoglycemia as the possible cause. In this patient, his chronic alcoholism and possible alcoholic liver disease are both potential causes of hypoglycemia. (D) Prostatism is unrelated to hypoglycemia. It often causes increased frequency in urination due to incomplete emptying of the urinary bladder due to a partial blockage of the urinary tract from an enlarged prostate gland. Because of increased urinary frequency, patients may initially fear that they have diabetes but are reassured by normal results on a finger-stick test or blood sugar evaluation.

454. **The answer is D.** (Caroline/Little Brown, *Unconscious States.*) (D) is correct, and the elevation in serum potassium level is due to the severity of the acidosis. This hyperkalemia may produce dangerous cardiac arrhythmias. As a result, some medical control physicians would recommend the administration of IV sodium bicarbonate in order to begin to correct the severe acidosis.

455. **The answer is D.** (Brady, *Endocrine and Metabolic Emergencies.*) (D) is correct. Since the patient is conscious and you suspect that this diabetic's bizarre behavior may be due to hypoglycemia, the treatment of choice is the oral administration of a glucose-containing substance. (A) is incorrect because, as long as the patient is able to take glucose by mouth, the correct route of administration is oral, not IV. (B) is not the first step in treatment. (C) is incorrect because the heart rate of 150 beats minute is probably a sinus tachycardia due to an acute hypoglycemic episode. The treatment of choice is to resolve the hypoglycemia, which will resolve the sinus tachycardia.

456. **The answer is C.** (Mosby, *Diabetic Emergencies.*) (A), (B), and (D) are correct. (C) is incorrect because, in hyperosmolar hyperglycemic nonketotic coma, there is no production of ketones and acids and no acidosis; therefore, there is no need to hyperventilate. Hyperventilation would be used to attempt to compensate for a metabolic acidosis.

457. **The answer is A.** (Brady, *Endocrine and Metabolic Emergencies.*) (B), (C), (D), insomnia, and fatigue are all signs or symptoms of hyperthyroidism. (A) is incorrect because with hyperthyroidism the patient has heat intolerance. A patient who is hypothyroid (underactive thyroid) has cold intolerance.

458. **The answer is D.** (Brady, *Endocrine and Metabolic Disorders.*) (A), (B), (C), weakness, and facial bloating are all signs and symptoms of hypothyroidism. (D) is incorrect because the hypothyroid patient has oily skin and hair.

459. **The answer is C.** (Mosby/ACEP, *Conditions by Diagnosis.*) (A), (B), (D), and rapid transport are the basic foundation of the prehospital emergent treatment of hyper- or hypothyroidism. At the emergency department, the severity of the thyroid disease will dictate the specific treatment of the over- or underactive thyroid gland. (C) is incorrect because usually the treatment of the over- or underactive thyroid gland will resolve most tachy- or bradyarrhythmias. Some hyperthyroid patients will present with atrial fibrillation with a rapid ventricular response. The treatment of choice is usually intravenous beta-blockers, such as IV propanolol (Inderal) or metoprolol (Lopressor), not digoxin.

460. **The answer is C.** (Brady, *Endocrine and Metabolic Emergencies.*) (A), (B), and (D) are correct. (C) is incorrect because an overactive adrenal gland produces hypokalemia (low potassium level).

461. **The answer is A.** (Mosby/ACEP, *Conditions by Diagnosis.*) (B), (C), (D), weight loss, and hypotension are frequent presenting signs and symptoms of adrenal gland hypofunction. (C) is incorrect because the adrenal gland normally produces and secretes epinephrine and norepinephrine. Adrenal gland hypofunction would produce less of these two essential hormones, resulting in hypotension. On the other hand, an overactive adrenal gland, known as Cushing's syndrome, frequently produces an excess of these two hormones, resulting in hypertension.

ANAPHYLAXIS

Directions: Each item below contains four suggested responses. Select the **one best** response to each item.

462. A hypersensitivity response to an allergen to which an organism has previously been exposed and to which the organism has developed antibodies is the definition of
(A) asthma
(B) allergic reaction
(C) a panic attack
(D) peripheral neuropathy

463. An acute, generalized, and violent antigen-antibody reaction, the most severe allergic reaction, which may be rapidly fatal, even with prompt and appropriate emergency medical care, is the definition of

(A) cardiac arrest
(B) urticaria
(C) anaphylaxis
(D) status epilepticus

464. An allergic reaction and/or an anaphylactic reaction is usually initiated after the body is exposed to

(A) an antibody
(B) a medication
(C) a bacteria
(D) an antigen

465. During an allergic and/or anaphylactic reaction, the mast cells and basophils produce a number of chemical mediators. The principal chemical mediator released is

(A) histamine
(B) epinephrine
(C) norepinephrine
(D) insulin

466. During an anaphylactic reaction, histamine produces all of the following effects EXCEPT

(A) vascular permeability, causing dilation of capillaries and venules
(B) contraction of coronary arteries
(C) contraction of smooth muscle, especially in the gastrointestinal tract and bronchi
(D) increase in gastric, nasal, and lacrimal secretions

467. All of the following are agents that may cause anaphylaxis EXCEPT

(A) antibiotics, bee stings, and aspirin
(B) nuts, eggs, and seafood
(C) nonsteroidal anti-inflammatory agents, aspirin, and x-ray contrast material
(D) water, Vaseline, and air

468. You are called to a holiday party for a 54-year-old female who is complaining of having eaten some fish with a fine gravy that contained some crushed almond nuts. Within 30 seconds, the patient complained of itching, hives, hoarseness, wheezing, dizziness, headache, nausea, vomiting, and diarrhea. In performing your assessment of this patient, all of the following are consistent with an allergic reaction or anaphylaxis EXCEPT

(A) a pulse rate of 34 beats per minute
(B) hives
(C) nausea, vomiting, and diarrhea
(D) hoarseness and wheezing

469. As you and your partner are cruising along a road by the beach, a frantic teenage boy is waving you down. He is screaming that a friend of his just got stung by a bee and is having difficulty breathing. As you approach this patient, you would expect all of the following possibilities EXCEPT

(A) patient's stating that he feels as if he is going to die
(B) swelling of the lips, tongue, and eyelids
(C) gangrene of the toes of the left foot
(D) chest tightness and wheezing

470. Which of the following is a very unusual manner in which an allergen gains access to the body and causes an anaphylactic reaction?

(A) injection by a needle or bee sting
(B) ingestion
(C) inhalation
(D) absorption across the skin

471. All of the following are signs or symptoms of anaphylaxis, rather than an allergic reaction, EXCEPT

(A) hoarseness and stridor
(B) hives and itching
(C) hypotension
(D) confusion and headache

472. You arrive at a private physician's office in your community for a 21-year-old male who has had an allergic reaction to an injection of penicillin. Upon your arrival, the nurse tells you that the patient had a strep throat and was given an intramuscular injection of penicillin about 15 minutes ago. Then, about 5 minutes ago, he began to complain about itchiness of the throat and swelling of the tongue. The doctor gave the patient an intramuscular injection of 50 mg Benadryl, but the patient then began to complain of hoarseness and having difficulty taking in air. As you walk into the examining room, you see a young man who is stridorous and in acute respiratory distress, breathing at 36 respirations per minute. His physical assessment revealed blood pressure of 124/78; pulse of 124 beats per minute; a large, swollen tongue; loud wheezing on lung examination; and several widespread hives. Which of the following is the first priority in the emergent treatment of this patient?

(A) ECG monitoring
(B) pulse oximetry
(C) 2 liters of Ringer's lactate solution wide open
(D) establishment and maintenance of the airway

473. In the patient presented in question 472, which would be the correct way to establish and maintain an airway?

(A) immediate cricothyrotomy
(B) blind insertion of an oropharyngeal airway
(C) oral endotracheal intubation
(D) oral tongue blade–guided insertion of an oropharyngeal airway

474. You are dispatched to a 65-year-old female who has taken a neighbor's prescription for a pain medication for arthritis. The patient admits to having two very dangerous reactions to Motrin and has been told to avoid medications in the same category. However, her neighbor's pain medication is Naprosyn, another nonsteroidal medication, like Motrin. After taking the medication, the patient noticed within 20 minutes that she became very itchy, with hives and an upset stomach. Over the past hour, the patient complains of weakness, dizziness and inability to walk for fear of falling. Your assessment reveals a flushed female who appears very weak, with a blood pressure of 70/46 supine and only palpable with sitting up. The patient otherwise shows diffuse hives, facial flushing, with clear lungs and a clear oral airway. After ensuring an open airway, all of the following are a part of the emergency care of this patient EXCEPT

(A) administration of 100 percent oxygen by nonrebreather mask
(B) 0.3 to 0.5 mg of 1:1000 epinephrine IV push
(C) large-bore IV line, with Ringer's lactate, to run wide open
(D) slow IV infusion of 5 to 10 mL of 1:10,000 epinephrine

475. In addition to the emergency care outlined in the above questions, all of the following are additional treatment options for a patient with anaphylaxis EXCEPT

    (A) diphenhydramine (Benadryl) 25 to 50 mg intramuscular or slow IV push

    (B) IV steroids (solumedrol or hydrocortisone)

    (C) inhaled beta agonists

    (D) IV beta blockers

476. Match all of the following medications used in the treatment of anaphylaxis, with the correct dosage:

    (A) epinephrine SC

    (B) epinephrine IV

    (C) Benadryl

    (D) Solumedrol

    (E) aminophylline

    (F) beta-agonist inhaler

    1. 25 to 50 mg

    2. 0.3 to 0.5 mg of 1:10,000

    3. 125 to 250 mg

    4. 2.5 mg in 3.0 mL normal saline solution

    5. 5.0 mg/kg loading dose

    6. 0.3 to 0.5 mg of 1:1000

477. You are dispatched to a 52-year-old male at an outpatient radiology center who has been injected with IV iodine in order to undergo an intravenous pyelogram to diagnose a possible kidney stone. The nursing staff notes that the patient was given an injection of iodine and, within 30 seconds, broke out in hives and complained of difficulty breathing. As you go into the examining room, you note that the patient is lying down. He is breathing at 26 breaths per minute and is able to speak clearly. His other vital signs are a normal temperature of 98° F, a blood pressure of 106/74, a regular pulse of 102 beats per minute, and a pulse oximetric measurement of 96 percent. Your assessment reveals a frightened male with bilateral diffuse wheezes, normal heart sounds, a soft abdomen with normal bowel sounds, grossly normal neurologic findings, and diffuse hives on the skin. After confirming a patent airway and initiating oxygen by nonrebreather mask, which is the first medication you should administer?

    (A) IV Solumedrol 125 mg

    (B) SC epinephrine 0.3 to 0.5 mg 1:1000 solution

    (C) Benadryl 25 to 50 mg

    (D) albuterol 2.5 mg in 3.0 mL of normal saline solution

ANAPHYLAXIS

A N S W E R S

462. The answer is B. (Mosby/ACEP, *Glossary.*) (B) is correct. (A) is incorrect because asthma is a chronic inflammatory disorder of the airways that is often aggravated by infections, stress, and certain allergens. (C) and (D) are unrelated to the definition.

463. The answer is C. (Brady, *Anaphylaxis.*) (C) is correct. (A) is incorrect because most cardiac arrests are unrelated to allergic reactions, even though an anaphylaxis patient may end up in cardiac arrest. (B) is a mild allergic reaction known as hives. (D) is due to epileptic seizure activity and is not an allergic reaction.

464. The answer is D. (Brady, *Anaphylaxis.*) (D) is correct. The antigen is usually some form of protein that causes the allergic patient's body to produce antibodies, usually IgE antibodies. These IgE antibodies become attached to the membranes of basophils and mast cells. (A) is incorrect because the antigen causes the allergic patient's body to produce antibody, not vice versa. (B) is one of many substances that act as an antigen and can produce an allergic and/or anaphylactic reaction. (C) is incorrect.

465. The answer is A. (Brady, *Anaphylaxis.*) (A) is correct. (B), (C), and (D) are incorrect because they are hormones, not chemical mediators.

466. The answer is B. (Mosby, *Anaphylaxis.*) (A), (C), and (D) are correct. (B) is incorrect, since there is no direct effect on the coronary arteries.

467. The answer is D. (Brady, *Anaphylaxis.*) (A), (B), (C), other medications, foreign proteins, wasps and other Hymenoptera stings, hormones (e.g., insulin), blood products, preservatives, and dextran are some of the agents that may cause anaphylaxis. (D) is incorrect because these substances usually do not produce anaphylaxis.

468. **The answer is A.** (Brady, *Anaphylaxis.*) (B), (C), and (D) are possibly present during an allergic or anaphylactic reaction. (A) is incorrect because most patients are tachycardic with an allergic reaction or anaphylaxis.

469. **The answer is C.** (Caroline/Little Brown, *Anaphylaxis.*) (A), (B), and (D) are correct. (C) is incorrect because gangrene is caused by a lack of arterial circulation over a prolonged period of time and is never an immediate reaction to an allergen.

470. **The answer is C.** (Caroline/Little Brown, *Anaphylaxis.*) (C) is correct. (A), (B), and (D) are incorrect because they are common methods of access for an allergen to the body, resulting in an anaphylactic reaction.

471. **The answer is B.** (Caroline/Little Brown, *Anaphylaxis.*) (A), (C), and (D) are correct. (B) may be seen with both an allergic reaction and an anaphylactic reaction.

472. **The answer is D.** (Caroline/Little Brown, *Anaphylaxis.*) (D) is truly the first priority in a patient having an anaphylactic reaction, which is manifested with stridor and threatening the upper airway. (A) and (B) are incorrect, even though of secondary importance in this patient. (C) is incorrect because this would be used for the anaphylactic patient who is demonstrating hypotension.

473. **The answer is C.** (Caroline/Little Brown, *Anaphylaxis.*) (C) is correct because this patient, with difficulty breathing, stridor, tachypnea, and a swollen tongue, has a jeopardized airway, and oral endotracheal intubation is the best method not only to establish but also to maintain the airway. (A) is incorrect because a needle cricothyrotomy is usually indicated for complete upper airway obstruction. If this patient's airway is unable to be maintained, he may soon become totally obstructed and require a needle cricothyrotomy. (B) and (D) are incorrect because, with stridor and a swollen tongue, insertion of an oropharyngeal airway may change this obstruction from a partial to a complete one.

474. **The answer is B.** (Caroline/Little Brown, *Anaphylaxis*; Brady, *Anaphylaxis.*) (A), (C), and (D) are correct. (B) is incorrect because 0.3 to 0.5 mg of 1:1000 is the correct dose of SC, not IV, epinephrine. This is the first line of epinephrine treatment in this patient. However, in a severe anaphylactic reaction, medical control may give permission for the administration of 5 to 10 mL (0.1 mL/kg) of 1:10,000 epinephrine by slow IV push.

475. **The answer is D.** (Brady, *Anaphylaxis*; Caroline/Little Brown, *Anaphylaxis.*) (D) is incorrect because IV beta blockers are not a part of the treatment of anaphylaxis and would be harmful in this situation. (A), (B), and (C) are other correct treatment options for anaphylaxis.

476. Answers. (Brady, *Anaphylaxis*; Caroline/Little Brown, *Anaphylaxis*.)
- (A) 6
- (B) 2
- (C) 1
- (D) 3
- (E) 5
- (F) 4

477. The answer is B. (Brady, *Anaphylaxis*.) (B) is correct because epinephrine is the treatment of choice for anaphylaxis. (A) is incorrect because this is a corticosteroid that may be an important part of the treatment of anaphylaxis, but not in the initial stage. (C) is used in the initial stage, but not before epinephrine. (D) is incorrect because it is appropriate for every patient with allergic wheezing, but in the patient with anaphylaxis, not before the administration of epinephrine.

GASTROENTEROLOGY

Directions: Each item below contains four suggested responses. Select the **one best** response to each item.

478. The intrathoracic abdomen includes all of the following EXCEPT

(A) kidneys
(B) stomach
(C) liver
(D) spleen

479. All of the following are classified as hollow abdominal organs EXCEPT

(A) stomach
(B) urinary bladder
(C) gallbladder
(D) spleen

480. The stretching of the autonomic nerve fibers that surround abdominal organs is known as

(A) somatic pain
(B) visceral pain
(C) referred pain
(D) cephalic pain

481. Irritation of the nerve fibers in the peritoneum by chemical or bacterial inflammation is known as

(A) visceral pain
(B) somatic pain
(C) cephalic pain
(D) referred pain

482. Pain that is felt in an area that is removed from the diseased organ is known as

(A) visceral pain
(B) referred pain
(C) somatic pain
(D) cervical pain

483. In obtaining a history from a patient with abdominal pain, the key points to be defined are represented by the letters PQRST. All of the following are matched with the correct definition EXCEPT

(A) P = provocative
(B) Q = quantity
(C) R = region
(D) T = timing

484. In the prehospital setting, all of the following are parts of the abdominal examination of the patient complaining of abdominal pain EXCEPT

(A) inspection
(B) auscultation for bowel sounds
(C) palpation
(D) determination of vital signs

485. You are dispatched to a 68-year-old female with acute abdominal pain. As you arrive at this patient's home, the patient admits to having a long-standing history of arthritis, which she self-medicates with Advil and aspirin. She notes that the arthritis has been particularly painful for the past 4 weeks, and she states that she has increased the use of both of these medications. The patient notes that her pain has been in the epigastric area for the past 5 days and that it is a burning pain associated with belching and vomiting. Your physical assessment reveals vital signs as follows: blood pressure 146/82, pulse 110 beats per minute, respirations 20 per minute. The patient is pale and diaphoretic and appears to be in mild distress. The abdominal examination reveals a nondistended abdomen, active bowel sounds, and epigastric tenderness without guarding or rebound. This presentation best represents which of the following diagnoses?

(A) bowel obstruction
(B) acute gastrointestinal bleeding
(C) acute gastritis
(D) acute kidney stone

486. As you drive to get gas, you are waved down by a frantic child, who states that his mother is having terrible stomach pains and needs help right away. As you run up the stairs to the patient's apartment, you find a 38-year-old female moaning in bed. She slowly explains that the pain started early this morning, with pain around the umbilicus associated with a lack of appetite, nausea, and constipation. During the day, the pain began to localize in the right lower quadrant. Upon assessment, the vital signs are blood pressure 100/72, pulse 112 per minute, and respirations 16 breaths per minute. Your abdominal examination reveals absent bowel sounds and marked right lower quadrant tenderness. The patient grabs your hand upon examination (guarding), and there is rebound tenderness as well. This acute abdominal emergency best represents which of the following diagnoses?

(A) acute duodenal ulcer
(B) acute appendicitis
(C) acute dysentery
(D) acute cholecystitis

487. In the questions 485 and 486, the acute prehospital management of the acute abdomen includes all of the following EXCEPT

(A) high-concentration oxygen
(B) IV saline solution or Ringer's lactate
(C) repeat abdominal examinations prior to transport
(D) immediate transport

488. As you arrive at the home of an 86-year-old male with abdominal pain, you request a history from the patient. He states that he has had left lower quadrant abdominal pain for over a week. However, only this morning the patient had the sudden onset of intense generalized abdominal pain, which intensifies with deep inspirations. Your assessment reveals the following vital signs: blood pressure 90/50, pulse 110 beats per minute, respiration 14 breaths per minute, and hot to touch. The abdominal examination reveals a distended abdomen without bowel sounds that is rigid and boardlike to palpation, with diffuse guarding and rebound. This case presentation best represents which of the following diagnoses?

(A) acute gastrointestinal bleeding
(B) acute appendicitis
(C) acute hepatitis
(D) perforated abdominal viscus

489. All of the following are signs or symptoms of acute upper gastrointestinal bleeding EXCEPT

(A) hematemesis
(B) pain in the epigastric or left upper quadrant, if present
(C) bleeding only with defecation
(D) dark stools, or melena

490. Match the following causes of upper gastrointestinal bleeding with the correct pathophysiology.

(A) gastritis
(B) bleeding esophageal varices
(C) gastric ulcer
(D) Mallory-Weiss tear
(E) duodenal ulcer
(F) esophagitis

1. eroding ulcer in the stomach
2. esophageal inflammation and erosions
3. diffuse inflammation in the stomach
4. eroding ulcer in the duodenum
5. bleeding, swollen esophageal veins
6. esophageal injury due to recurrent vomiting

491. You are dispatched to a 74-year-old female who is vomiting blood. Upon your arrival at the patient's home, you notice four large pans filled with blood and mucus. The patient states that she has arthritis and has been getting progressively worse. Under her doctor's direction, she has been taking increasing amounts of Advil and aspirin. In the past week, she has taken two tablets of 200-mg Advil five times per day and two aspirins two to three times a day as well. She has been having stomach pains, nausea, and anorexia over this same period of time but just this morning began to vomit. Initially, the vomit was only blood streaked; however, since noon it has been almost entirely bright-red blood. Your initial assessment reveals that the patient is afebrile and has the following vital signs: respiratory rate 16 breaths per minute, pulse 112 beats per minute lying supine and 130 beats per minute sitting upright, and blood pressure 90/62 lying supine and 60 palpable sitting upright. All of the following are part of the prehospital emergency care of the patient suffering from acute upper gastrointestinal bleeding EXCEPT

(A) high-concentration oxygen
(B) securing a patent airway
(C) initiating blood transfusions
(D) starting two large-bore IV sites and beginning to administer Ringer's lactate or normal saline solution

492. Which of the following is the best definition of lower gastrointestinal bleeding?

   (A) left lower abdominal pain
   (B) bright-red blood or wine-colored bleeding per rectum
   (C) vomiting blood with lower abdominal pain
   (D) urinating blood

493. Match the following causes of lower gastrointestinal hemorrhage with the correct pathophysiology.

   (A) diverticulosis
   (B) arteriovenous malformations
   (C) colon carcinoma or tumor
   (D) rectal fissures
   (E) hemorrhoids
   (F) inflammatory bowel disease

   1. external and/or internal bleeding rectal veins
   2. vascular abnormalities, frequently in right colon
   3. ulcerations and erythema of colon and/or small bowel
   4. bleeding diverticuli of the colon
   5. cracks in the rectal tissue
   6. abnormal growths in colon

494. You are assigned to an 85-year-old male with rectal bleeding. As you enter the patient's bedroom, you find the patient appearing weak and pale, with blood and clots in the sheets. The patient denies having previous episodes of rectal bleeding. As you begin to assess the patient, you find that the patient's vital signs are respiratory rate 16 breaths per minute, pulse 112 beats per minute supine and 140 breaths per minute sitting up, and blood pressure 94 supine and 70 palpable sitting up. The abdominal examination reveals a nondistended abdomen that is soft, and nontender, with active bowel sounds. The prehospital treatment of a lower gastrointestinal hemorrhage includes all of the following EXCEPT

   (A) 100 percent oxygen
   (B) IV line with saline lock KVO (keep vein open)
   (C) ECG monitoring
   (D) rapid transport

495. You are assigned to an 84-year-old female nursing home resident for stomach upset. As you arrive at the patient's bedside, she admits to a 3-day history of feeling sick with nausea, vomiting, and occasional watery diarrhea associated with mild abdominal cramps. The patient felt sick but was still able to ambulate and take care of her daily activities. The patient stated that everyone at the nursing home was worried about her inability to keep food down. Your physical assessment reveals that the patient's vital signs are blood pressure 118/74 without postural changes, pulse 86 beats per minute, and respirations 16 breaths per minute. The patient's abdomen is soft and nontender, with active bowel sounds. Which of the following best represents the cause of this patient's problem?

(A) acute gastrointestinal hemorrhage
(B) acute appendicitis
(C) acute gastroenteritis
(D) ulcerative colitis

496. Match each of the following conditions with the correct pathophysiology.

(A) diverticulitis
(B) appendicitis
(C) intestinal obstruction
(D) peptic ulcer disease
(E) pancreatitis
(F) Crohn's disease

1. inflammation of tissue at tip of the cecum
2. inflammation of an epigastric organ caused by trauma, alcohol, drugs, and so on
3. ulceration, edema, and erythema of the small intestine and colon
4. ulceration, edema, and erythema of stomach and/or duodenum
5. blockage of the movement of intestinal contents due to adhesions, tumor, hernia, fecal impaction, and other conditions
6. inflammation of pockets off the colon

497. You are dispatched to a nursing home for a " sick and jaundiced" 76-year-old male. As you arrive at the home, the nurse in charge rushes to tell you that this is the third patient in the past week with the same type of illness. This patient complains of 4 to 5 days of feeling very tired, with darkening of urine; light, clay-colored stools; dull, right upper quadrant pain; and loss of appetite. Your physical examination reveals a blood pressure of 128/72, respirations of 14 breaths per minute, a pulse of 74 beats per minute, yellow sclera, yellow skin, clear lungs, and a nondistended, soft abdomen with active bowel sounds and mild right upper quadrant tenderness without guarding and without rebound tenderness. As you discuss the approach to treating this patient with your partner, which of the following is most important in preventing any possible spread of this condition?

(A) Request vaccination of all the nursing home residents.
(B) Draw blood work to specifically define the type of disease.
(C) Use body-substance isolation precautions.
(D) Carefully collect all vomitus and stool-stained sheets and clothing.

498. You are assigned to a 38-year-old female with abdominal pain. You arrive at the patient's home and find the patient lying in bed in acute pain. The patient notes that, for the past 12 hours, she has had recurrent episodes of severe epigastric and right upper quadrant pain that is severe and associated with nausea, vomiting, and shaking chills. Your assessment reveals a blood pressure of 112/72, respirations of 12 breaths per minute, a pulse of 90 beats per minute, and a slightly distended abdomen with active bowel sounds and marked right upper quadrant tenderness without guarding or rebound. All of the following are correct statements concerning this patient's illness EXCEPT

(A) The pain is often precipitated by fatty foods.
(B) It should be treated with IV fluids.
(C) There is often a patient and/or family history of gallstones.
(D) Prehospital treatment may include IV narcotics for pain control.

GASTROENTEROLOGY

478. The answer is A. (Caroline/Little Brown, *Acute Abdomen.*) (A) is incorrect because the kidneys are located in the retroperitoneum. (B), (C), and (D) are correct because the lower ribs of the thoracic ribcage cover them all.

479. The answer is D. (Caroline/Little Brown, *Acute Abdomen.*) (D) is a solid abdominal organ, along with the liver, kidneys, pancreas, and the ovaries. (A), (B), (C), the small and large bowel, and the uterus are all hollow abdominal organs.

480. The answer is B. (Caroline/Little Brown, *Acute Abdomen.*) (B) is correct. It is noted as being diffuse and poorly localized pain, often accompanied by nausea, vomiting, sweating, and tachycardia. (A), (C), and (D) are all incorrect.

481. The answer is B. (Caroline/Little Brown, *Acute Abdomen.*) (B) is correct and is more localized than visceral pain, sharp, constant, and often worsened by coughing or jarring movements. (A), (C), and (D) are incorrect.

482. The answer is B. (Caroline/Little Brown, *Acute Abdomen.*) (B) is correct, and an example is when a kidney stone, which is lodged in the ureter, causes pain that usually radiates down the inner thigh and into the genitalia. (A), (C), and (D) are all incorrect.

483. The answer is B. (Brady, *Gastrointestinal, Genitourinary, and Reproductive Emergencies*; Caroline/Little Brown, *Acute Abdomen.*) (A), (C), and (D) are correct. S stands for severity, and Q stands for quality. Some texts precede PQRST with the letter O, which stands for onset. Others add the suffix letter A, which stands for associated symptoms. (B) is incorrect because Q stands for quality, not quantity.

484. **The answer is B.** (Brady, *Gastrointestinal, Genitourinary, and Reproductive Emergencies*; Caroline/Little Brown, *Acute Abdomen.*) (A), (C), and (D) are the key parts of the abdominal examination. (B) is incorrect because most texts note that it is extremely difficult to perform auscultation of the abdomen in the prehospital setting because of the outside noise interference.

485. **The answer is C.** (Brady, *Gastrointestinal, Genitourinary, and Reproductive Emergencies.*) (C) is correct. (A) is incorrect because it is often associated with severe constipation, abdominal distention, and, often, absent bowel sounds. (B) is incorrect because the patient is not vomiting blood and does not have melena (black bowel movements). (D) is incorrect because a patient usually complains of pain on one side, with colicky spasms.

486. **The answer is B.** (Mosby, *Acute Abdominal Pain and Renal Failure.*) (B) is correct. (A) is incorrect because usually acute duodenal ulcer pain presents as upper abdominal pain, sometimes with vomiting with or without blood, associated with epigastric or right upper abdominal focal tenderness. (C) is incorrect because it usually presents with recurrent bouts of diarrhea. (D) is incorrect because cholecystitis represents an acutely inflamed gallbladder, which usually includes belching, flatus, and right upper abdominal pain sometimes radiating to the back and shoulder, and right upper abdominal tenderness, sometimes with guarding and rebound.

487. **The answer is C.** (Brady, *Gastrointestinal, Genitourinary, and Reproductive Emergencies.*) (A), (B), (D), keeping the patient supine, and monitoring vital signs and cardiac rhythm are all part of the prehospital emergency management. (C) is incorrect because, since the treatment of the acute abdomen is often a surgical emergency, there should not be any delay in transport to the emergency department.

488. **The answer is D.** (Brady, *Gastrointestinal, Genitourinary, and Reproductive Emergencies.*) (D) is correct and may be caused by various conditions, such as a diverticulum of the colon, a ruptured appendix, or a perforated duodenal or gastric ulcer. (A) is incorrect because of a lack of vomiting blood or melena (black tarry stools). (B) is incorrect because of an absence of periumbilical pain or right lower quadrant pain, nausea, lack of appetite, and right lower quadrant tenderness. (C) is incorrect because there is usually a history of fatigue, yellow jaundice, dark urine, and light stools, and the physical examination usually only shows right upper quadrant tenderness.

489. **The answer is C.** (Brady, *Gastrointestinal, Genitourinary, and Reproductive Emergencies.*) (A), (B), and (D) are correct. (C) is incorrect because it is usually a sign of rectal bleeding from hemorrhoids, tumor, and so on.

490. Answers. (Mosby/ACEP, *Gastrointestinal Conditions.*)
- (A) 3
- (B) 5
- (C) 1
- (D) 6
- (E) 4
- (F) 2

491. The answer is C. (Mosby, *Acute Abdominal Pain and Renal Failure;* Mosby/ACEP, *Gastrointestinal Conditions.*) (A), (B), (D), ECG monitoring, and rapid transport are all parts of the emergency care. (C) is incorrect because initiating blood transfusions is part of the care in the emergency department, not in the prehospital setting. The only exception is for a patient requiring extrication who receives blood transfusions while awaiting extrication.

492. The answer is B. (Mosby/ACEP, *Gastrointestinal, Genitourinary, and Reproductive Emergencies.*) (B) is the correct definition. (A) is incorrect because left lower abdominal pain is usually not accompanied by any gastrointestinal bleeding. (C) is incorrect because upper gastrointestinal bleeding is defined by vomiting blood. (D) is incorrect because urinating blood is known as hematuria.

493. Answers. (Mosby/ACEP, *Gastrointestinal Conditions;* Mosby, *Acute Abdominal Pain and Renal Failure.*)
- (A) 4
- (B) 2
- (C) 6
- (D) 5
- (E) 1
- (F) 3

494. The answer is B. (Mosby/ACEP, *Gastrointestinal Conditions.*) (A), (C), and (D) are correct. (B) is incorrect because, with a lower (or upper) gastrointestinal hemorrhage, the correct IV fluid of choice is two IV lines of Ringer's lactate or normal saline solution. An IV KVO is incorrect, particularly in this patient, who has postural hypotension from lower gastrointestinal hemorrhage. This patient requires aggressive IV fluid administration.

495. The answer is C. (Mosby/ACEP, *Gastrointestinal Conditions.*) (C) is correct. (A) is incorrect because there is no history or evidence of any hematemesis or melena. (B) is incorrect because there is no evidence of periumbilical or right lower quadrant pain or right lower quadrant tenderness. (D) is incorrect because there is no evidence of bloody, mucousy diarrhea.

496. Answers. (Mosby/ACEP, *Gastrointestinal Conditions.*)

   (A) 6

   (B) 1

   (C) 5

   (D) 4

   (E) 2

   (F) 3

497. The answer is C. (Mosby/ACEP, *Gastrointestinal Conditions*; Brady, *Gastrointestinal, Genitourinary, and Reproductive Emergencies.*) (C) is correct because it will help to prevent further spread of this outbreak of viral hepatitis. (A) is incorrect because body-substance isolation precautions are the most important steps in preventing the spread of an outbreak of viral hepatitis. Vaccinations may play a role in further limiting the spread of an outbreak. (B) is incorrect because blood work may further define the precise cause of such an outbreak but will not immediately prevent further spread of the hepatitis outbreak. (D) is incorrect because, without body-substance isolation precautions, incorrectly collecting all of the vomitus and stool-stained sheets and clothing may actually cause further spread of the hepatitis to you and/or your partner and the personnel in the laundry.

498. The answer is D. (Mosby, *Acute Abdominal Pain and Renal Failure.*) (A), (B), and (C) are correct. (D) is incorrect because all patients with acute abdominal pain, from any number of causes, should never be treated with narcotics, which may relieve the pain but hide the seriousness of the disease and prevent the rapid identification of the cause. This may also delay the emergent treatment of the problem.

RENAL AND UROLOGY

Directions: Each item below contains four suggested responses. Select the **one best** response to each item.

499. Which of the following is the best definition of acute renal failure?

(A) difficulty in passing urine
(B) patient on renal dialysis machine with difficulty breathing
(C) rapid and potentially reversible deterioration of kidney function
(D) acute urinary tract infection with difficulty urinating

500. Which of the following is the correct sequence for the flow of urine through the renal and urinary system?

(A) Ureters, kidneys, bladder, urethra
(B) Bladder, kidneys, urethra, ureters
(C) Kidneys, ureters, bladder, urethra
(D) Ureters, bladder, urethra, kidneys

501. All of the following are various presentations of common acute urinary disorders EXCEPT

(A) urinary tract infection
(B) urinary retention
(C) urinary alkalosis
(D) urinary stones

502. All of the following are mechanisms for the development of acute renal failure EXCEPT

(A) prerenal: shock and dehydration
(B) renal: trauma, nephrotoxic drugs, or kidney infection
(C) postrenal: obstruction of the urinary flow
(D) urinary tract infection

503. You are dispatched to a 76-year-old "sick" male. Upon questioning the patient and his family, you are told that he has a long-standing history of difficulty urinating and getting up to urinate several times at night. However, in the past 3 to 4 days, the patient's wife noted that he developed a high fever but strangely was not going to the bathroom and yet was not incontinent of urine on his clothes or in the bed. Now, in the past 3 hours, he has been moaning and is less coherent. Your physical assessment reveals a blood pressure of 98/72, respirations of 20 breaths per minute, a pulse of 112 beats per minute, clear lungs, normal heart sounds, and a distended abdomen, active bowel sounds, and a palpable fullness in the lower abdomen. The most likely cause of this patient's problem is

(A) acute renal failure due to the ingestion of renal toxic medications
(B) acute renal failure due to a cancer of the kidney
(C) acute renal failure due to a kidney stone
(D) acute renal failure due to urinary output obstruction due to an enlarged prostate with a secondary infection

504. You arrive at the home of an 87-year-old female who has a history of "kidney problems" and is complaining of decreased urinary output, fatigue, loss of appetite, nausea, vomiting, and generalized swelling of her legs and abdomen. Your initial assessment reveals a blood pressure of 178/112, a pulse of 88 beats per minute, respirations of 26 breaths per minute, and pasty yellow skin and 4+ pitting leg edema. This patient's case best represents which of the following diagnoses?

(A) acute renal failure
(B) chronic renal failure
(C) acute urinary tract infection
(D) prostate cancer

505. Based on the case presentation in question 504, which of the following are the most probable blood work results in this patient with chronic renal failure?

(A) hyperkalemia and metabolic acidosis
(B) hypokalemia and metabolic alkalosis
(C) hypernatremia and polycythemia
(D) hypernatremia and normal serum creatinine

506. All of the following are possible nervous system presentations of chronic renal failure EXCEPT

(A) delirium
(B) seizures
(C) earache
(D) muscle twitching

507. Which of the following is the best definition of renal dialysis?

(A) process of using a programmable machine to assist in urinating for the patient
(B) process of passing a nasogastric tube in order to remove toxic ingestions
(C) process of providing antibiotics to an infected kidney(s) by way of an arterial catheter
(D) process of exchanging biochemical substances across a semipermeable membrane to remove toxic substances

508. All of the following are known complications of dialysis EXCEPT

(A) chest pain or dysrhythmia
(B) hypotension
(C) stomach ulcers
(D) disequilibrium syndrome

509. Which of the following is the best definition of renal calculi?

(A) kidney stones, the result of crystal aggregation in the kidney's collecting system
(B) the calculator component of a dialysis machine
(C) the formula used to calculate whether a patient is in kidney failure
(D) stones that form in other organs and result in damaging kidney function

510. You are dispatched to a 44-year-old male complaining of the acute onset, 1 hour ago, of severe pain in his right side. The patient states that he went to work this morning feeling fine and then suddenly felt an intense pain, which he rated as a 10 in severity. He stated that the pain was associated with nausea, and he even vomited once. After about 20 minutes, the pain suddenly resolved and he was joking with his coworkers that he must have had gas. Then, about 15 minutes later, the pain returned but was a little lower in his right side and seemed to spread into his right testicle. He noted that his testicle appeared normal and was not tender to touch. He again noted that the pain was very intense and was as painful as when he fractured his leg in a football game. Your physical assessment reveals a blood pressure of 146/88, a pulse of 94 beats per minute, respirations of 18 breaths per minute, active bowel sounds, a nondistended and nontender abdomen, and no guarding or rebound tenderness. Based on this patient's presentation, the key part of his emergent prehospital treatment would include which of the following?

(A) request for only IV morphine from medical control
(B) syrup of ipecac
(C) only nasal oxygen and ECG monitoring
(D) IV fluids

RENAL AND UROLOGY

A N S W E R S

499. The answer is C. (Brady, *Gastrointestinal, Genitourinary, and Reproductive Emergencies.*) (C) is correct. (A) is incorrect because difficulty urinating may be related to a urinary problem but is not a definition of acute renal failure. (B) is incorrect because difficulty breathing is not a specific sign of acute renal failure, especially in a patient with a known diagnosis of chronic renal failure. (D) is incorrect for the same reason as (A).

500. The answer is C. (Mosby, *Acute Abdominal Pain and Renal Failure.*) (C) is the correct sequence for urinary flow. (A), (B), and (D) are incorrect.

501. The answer is C. (Mosby, *Acute Abdominal Pain and Renal Failure.*) (A), (B), and (D) are all common acute urinary disorders. (C) is incorrect because there is no such condition as urinary alkalosis.

502. The answer is D. (Brady, *Gastrointestinal, Genitourinary, and Reproductive Emergencies.*) (A), (B), and (C) are the three mechanisms for the development of acute renal failure. (D) is incorrect because a urinary tract infection by itself does not cause acute renal failure.

503. The answer is D. (Brady, *Gastrointestinal, Genitourinary, and Reproductive Emergencies.*) (D) is correct, with total urinary tract obstruction due to an enlarged prostate, which has produced a distended urinary bladder, which appears as a lower abdominal midline mass. The development of fever may have represented an infection, which, if located in the kidneys may actually worsen the acute renal failure. (A) is incorrect because the ingestion of renal toxic medications should not produce urinary tract obstruction with a distended urinary bladder. (B) is incorrect because a kidney cancer should not lead to acute renal failure because it occurs in only one kidney and would produce acute renal failure only if the patient had only one kidney. (C) is incorrect because usually the patient begins by complaining of intense pain on one side of the back or flank. It also would only rarely produce a distended bladder, if a kidney stone became lodged in the urethra and totally blocked the outflow of urine.

504. **The answer is B.** (Mosby, *Acute Abdominal Pain and Renal Failure.*) (B) is correct because the patient is demonstrating the following signs of chronic renal failure: high blood pressure, pasty yellow skin with uremic white frost, decreased urinary output, marked pitting edema, pulmonary edema, and distended neck veins. Other consistent findings are anorexia, nausea, vomiting, and fatigue. (A) is incorrect because, although some of the findings may be present with acute or chronic failure, pulmonary edema and 4+ pitting edema of the legs and abdomen take time to develop. (C) is incorrect because an acute urinary tract infection simply produces frequent urination, dysuria, nocturia, and sometimes a low-grade fever. (D) is incorrect because it is anatomically impossible for a woman to get prostate cancer.

505. **The answer is A.** (Caroline/Little Brown, *Acute Abdomen.*) (A) is correct. Hyperkalemia is an increased serum potassium level, and metabolic acidosis is due to an accumulation of body acids. (B) is incorrect because hypokalemia means a low serum potassium level and metabolic alkalosis, which are usually not signs of chronic renal failure. (C) is incorrect because hypernatremia is an elevated serum sodium level, which is usually not present in the face of fluid overload from chronic renal failure. Polycythemia is represented by an increase in the red blood cell count, while chronic renal failure patients are usually chronically anemic. (D) is incorrect because of the reasons given in the previous discussion of hypernatremia and because patients with chronic renal insufficiency have marked elevations of both serum creatinine and blood urea nitrogen levels.

506. **The answer is C.** (Mosby, *Acute Andominal Pain and Renal Failure.*) (A), (B), (D), anxiety, obtundation, and hallucinations are some of the nervous system manifestations of chronic renal failure. (C) is not a sign of chronic renal failure.

507. **The answer is D.** (Brady, *Gastrointestinal, Genitourinary, and Reproductive Emergencies.*) (D) is correct. The two basic types are hemodialysis and peritoneal dialysis. (A) is incorrect because renal dialysis is unrelated to urination. (B) is incorrect because this process is known as gastric lavage. (C) is incorrect because renal dialysis is unrelated to the delivery of antibiotics by any mechanism.

508. **The answer is C.** (Brady, *Gastrointestinal, Genitourinary, and Reproductive Emergencies.*) (A), (B), (D), and air embolism are known complications of renal dialysis. (C) is incorrect because, even though sometimes chronic renal failure patients on dialysis may develop stomach upset with nausea and/or vomiting, this is not due to the development of stomach ulcers.

509. The answer is A. (Brady, *Gastrointestinal, Genitourinary, and Reproductive Emergencies.*) (A) is correct. (B) is incorrect because there is no such computer. (C) is incorrect because there is no such formula. (D) is incorrect because other stones, such as gallstones, are unrelated to the functioning of the kidney.

510. The answer is D. (Brady, *Gastrointestinal, Genitourinary, and Reproductive Emergencies.*) (D) is correct because this patient's presentation is classic for having "renal colic" due to a kidney stone lodged in his right renal collecting system (usually in the ureter). Administering IV fluids is a key part of treating this patient because it will increase the amount of urine produced by the kidney, which will help push the stone down the ureter and into the urinary bladder, which will immediately cause the pain to resolve. In the urinary bladder, the stone may dissolve, be passed out the urethra with urinating, or, rarely, become lodged in the urethra, where it can be extracted. (A) is incorrect because, although many prehospital protocols will permit Paramedics to administer analgesics in the field, it is not as important as providing IV fluids. (B) is incorrect because this presentation is not related to a drug or toxic ingestion, and syrup of ipecac has no role in the treatment of renal colic. (C) is incorrect because these are not a key part of the treatment of renal colic, even though they would be instituted in the overall care of this patient.

TOXICOLOGY

Directions: Each item below contains four suggested responses. Select the **one best** response to each item.

511. All of the following are routes of exposure for toxicologic emergencies EXCEPT

(A) ingestion
(B) surface absorption
(C) inhalation
(D) aspiration

512. Regional poison control centers are available for assisting in the treatment of toxicologic emergencies in all of the following manners EXCEPT

(A) They often are able to be contacted directly by emergency medical services providers.
(B) With their assistance, definitive care can often be initiated in the prehospital setting for over 8 percent of toxicologic emergencies.
(C) They will always dispatch personnel to the scene to assist with the emergent treatment of each acutely poisoned patient.
(D) They can help coordinate the treatment of the poisoned patient by calling ahead and notifying the receiving hospital while the ambulance is in route.

513. The total number of reported poisonings in the United States each year is approximately

(A) 150,000 patients
(B) 250,000 patients
(C) 575,000 patients
(D) 1,000,000 patients

514. Of the 1,000,000 poisonings, which is the correct percentage of cases occurring in children less than 5 years of age?

(A) 10%
(B) 25%
(C) 50%
(D) 75%

515. All of the following are contra-indications to inducing vomiting in the poisoned patient EXCEPT

(A) a seizing patient
(B) a patient with an acetaminophen (Tylenol) overdose
(C) a stuporous patient
(D) a pregnant patient

516. You are dispatched to the home of a 3-year-old boy who was found lying on the floor next to an empty bottle of adult acetaminophen (Tylenol) tablets. The patient's mother is very upset and states that she just bought the bottle of 100 tablets of 500-mg acetaminophen 4 days ago. She herself had taken 10 tablets in the past few days and had just taken 2 tablets a few hours ago and left the top off of the bottle when the telephone rang. Upon returning to the bedroom, she found her child chewing on a few tablets, with only 60 tablets remaining in the bottle. The child appears alert, is in no distress, and has stable vital signs and normal physical examination findings. When you call medical control, the telemetry physician wants you to begin to prevent the child from absorbing the acetaminophen. All of the following are prehospital emergency care treatment options for preventing absorption of an ingested poison EXCEPT

(A) Administer syrup of ipecac.
(B) Perform a colon lavage.
(C) Administer activated charcoal.
(D) Pass an orogastric tube to perform gastric lavage.

517. You are dispatched to a 4-year-old child who is having difficulty breathing. As you arrive at the house, the child's tearful father calls you into the kitchen. His son is sitting on the floor, complaining of a very sore throat. The child's father notes that he left him eating his cereal, while he took a shower and shaved, about 45 minutes ago. Upon returning, he found the child sitting on the floor with an open Drano container. The child readily admits swallowing three handfuls of the contents and is complaining of increasing throat pain. The patient's vital signs are blood pressure 96/62, pulse rate 110 beats per minute and regular, and respiratory rate 32 breaths per minute. The child is becoming hoarse, and his respiratory rate is continuing to rise to 40 breaths per minute. His mouth reveals small Drano particles and some redness and swelling. His chest is clear, but he is beginning to use his accessory muscles and has some nasal flaring. Which of the following is the top priority in caring for this child with a caustic ingestion?

(A) Administer syrup of ipecac.
(B) Perform gastric lavage.
(C) Immediately transport to the hospital with 100 percent oxygen and focusing on airway management with possible airway obstruction.
(D) Try to administer lemon juice or vinegar to neutralize this alkali ingestion.

518. You arrive at the apartment of an elderly female who states that she was babysitting her 3-year-old granddaughter today. About 15 minutes ago, she found the child crying in the dining room with an opened bottle of furniture polish. The child appears to have taken half of the bottle and is having obvious difficulty breathing, with a respiratory rate of 50 breaths per minute. At present, the child's airway is open, yet she is beginning to have increasing use of accessory muscles and central cyanosis. On physical examination, the child has diffuse rales and rhonchi. Which of the following is the first priority in providing emergency care to this child?

(A) administering nasal oxygen at 3 to 4 liters/minute
(B) calling medical control to discuss options for inducing vomiting
(C) administering IV morphine sulfate
(D) endotracheal intubation followed by administration of 100 percent oxygen

519. All of the following are true statements concerning toxic inhalations EXCEPT

(A) Carbon monoxide poisoning is a part of every toxic inhalation.
(B) Removal of the patient from the toxic environment is crucial.
(C) The Paramedic should not enter the toxic environment without protective breathing apparatus.
(D) Often there is more than one victim.

520. All of the following are causes of inhalation poisoning EXCEPT

(A) cyanide
(B) chlorine gas
(C) carbon monoxide
(D) aspirin

521. In the middle of winter, you are called to evaluate a 68-year-old man because he was found "acting bizarre." As you arrive at the patient's home, his wife hurriedly waves you into the house. She tells you that they have recently purchased this winter home, which had not been used for over 2 years. Her husband went into the basement to start up a small fireplace about 40 minutes ago. He had come up about 10 minutes ago, complaining of a headache. He was nauseous and actually vomited on the floor. Upon questioning him, she found that he was confused and did not make sense. Right after she called 911 for an ambulance, she returned to find her husband having a seizure, and then he became unresponsive. All of the following are parts of the emergency treatment options for this patient EXCEPT

(A) immediately removing the patient from the home
(B) assessing the ABCs and beginning to administer 100 percent oxygen
(C) contacting poison control or medical control to discuss the quickest means of transfer to a hyperbaric chamber
(D) immediately proceeding down to the basement to personally investigate the possible source of the problem

522. You are called to a home of a 14-year-old boy who is exhibiting bizarre behavior. As you arrive at the scene, you find the patient being surrounded by his family and acting upset and scared because of frightening hallucinations. As you are trying to calmly talk with and assess this emotionally disturbed patient, his 12-year-old brother states that the patient has "sniffed glue" in the past few weeks. All of the following are possible signs of inhalant abuse EXCEPT

(A) smell of a chemical solvent on the patient's breath
(B) diffuse red skin rash
(C) evidence of product containers or huffing or bagging paraphernalia
(D) glue or paint on the patient's hands, face, or clothes

523. All of the following are causes of injected poisoning EXCEPT

(A) dog bite
(B) bee sting
(C) spider bite
(D) wasp bite

524. You are dispatched to the county fair for a 6-year-old boy who has been stung by a bee. As you approach the crying child in his mother's arms, you notice that his right forearm is red and swollen at the site of the witnessed sting. You have determined that the child has only a localized reaction to the sting, with stable vital signs and no signs of anaphylaxis. As you begin to treat the bite site, you notice that the "stinger" is still present at the site. Which of the following is the correct way to remove the stinger?

(A) Gently squeeze two sides of the sting site and pull the stinger out.
(B) Use a forceps to pull it out.
(C) Use a scalpel blade to cut out the piece of skin containing the stinger.
(D) Using a scalpel or knife blade, carefully scrape the stinger and its sac from the wound.

525. You are dispatched to a 20-year-old with a spider bite. As you walk up to the patient, he explains that he went outside to the woodshed to get a few pieces of firewood. He initially thought that he saw a spider near the wood pile, but then it was gone. In proceeding to pick up a few logs, he felt a bite on his lower leg. When he looked down, he recognized a large black widow spider. As you begin to examine the patient, you think of the possible physical findings that may be caused by a black widow spider bite. All of the following are such findings EXCEPT

(A) immediate localized redness and swelling at the site of the bite
(B) progressive severe muscle spasms
(C) severe abdominal pain with lower-extremity bite
(D) gross hematuria

526. Which of the following is the best definition of drug overdose?

(A) taking prescription medications too rapidly
(B) refers only to taking "street" drugs
(C) a combination of normal doses of prescribed medications and a moderate amount of alcohol
(D) poisoning from a pharmacological substance, either legal or illegal

527. You are dispatched to a nearby college dormitory for an unresponsive 18-year-old male. As you arrive at his room, two students approach you and ask that you please keep the story they are about to tell confidential. Evidently, last night was initiation into their fraternity and the patient was one of the new pledges. As part of the ritual, he was made to drink several glasses of straight liquor, including Scotch, bourbon, gin, and others. As the night progressed, this young man became increasingly drunk, and so they simply escorted him to a bed in the fraternity house. However, when the fire alarm went off this morning, about 4 hours after he went to bed, he did not respond and was found unresponsive in bed. As you examine the patient, you note that he is truly unresponsive to painful stimuli, with midsize reactive pupils. His vital signs are a blood pressure of 88/64, a pulse of 114 beats per minute and regular, and respirations of 8 breaths per minute. In assessing his airway, you note the presence of alcoholic-smelling vomit in his mouth and on his face, gurgling respirations, and absence of a gag reflex. As a Paramedic, your emergency medical care should include all of the following EXCEPT

(A) oral suctioning
(B) endotracheal intubation
(C) IV thiamine, naloxone (Narcan), and $D_{50}W$
(D) syrup of ipecac

528. You respond to an "overdosed" 24-year-old female. As you enter the patient's apartment and approach the patient, you notice that the patient and her mother are crying. The patient's mother states that about a week ago, her daughter's boyfriend was returning home from law school to see her, when he had a fatal car accident. She has been distraught ever since and, according to her mother, very depressed. Today, after being out all day with some friends, the mother found the patient in her bedroom with an empty bottle of her phenobarbital (30-mg tablets), which she takes for a seizure disorder. Her mother states that she usually takes one tablet three times a day and just yesterday had received a new month's supply of 90 tablets. As you approach the patient, you notice that she appears to be in a drunken state, with slurred speech, and is falling asleep. The patient's initial vital signs include a pulse of 120 beats per minute, respirations of 18 breaths per minute, and a blood pressure of 90/64. She also has dilated pupils, clammy skin, and an intact gag reflex. All of the following are part of the Paramedic's emergency care for this patient EXCEPT

(A) IV thiamine, naloxone (Narcan), and $D_{50}W$
(B) syrup of ipecac
(C) activated charcoal
(D) IV fluids and ECG monitoring

529. In treating a patient with a cocaine overdose, all of the following medications may be given, if indicated, EXCEPT

(A) nitroglycerin for chest pain
(B) benzodiazepines, such as midazolam (Versed) or lorazepam (Ativan), for seizures
(C) IV lidocaine for ventricular tachycardia with a pulse
(D) IV flumazenil (Mazecon) for a concurrent diazepam (Valium) overdose

530. You are waved down at the site of one of the city's well-known "crack houses" by an upset 20-year-old female. She states that she and her boyfriend went inside to look for a friend, and then her boyfriend proceeded to try "a little" crack. Now she is very upset because he is inside acting very strange and appears very sick. As you enter the house accompanied by a police escort, you find a 24-year-old male sitting on an old couch, excited and appearing bizarre. All of the following are possible physical findings in a patient with a cocaine overdose EXCEPT

(A) euphoria, dilated pupils, and bradycardia
(B) twitching, anxiety, and psychosis
(C) tachycardia, somnolence, and hypertension
(D) hyperactivity, rapid and irregular pulse, and seizures

531. Match the following drugs with their "street" names.

(A) heroin _____
(B) barbiturates _____
(C) phencyclidine _____
(D) cocaine _____
(E) marijuana _____
(F) methaqualone (Quaalude) _____
(G) methadone _____
(H) amphetamines _____

1. bennies, black beauties, uppers
2. angel dust, loveboat, hog
3. lude, quay, soaps
4. snow, blow, white powder
5. horse, smack, antifreeze
6. dollies, dolls
7. blues, downs, downers
8. pot, reefer, weed

532. You are dispatched to a small, old hotel for a 58-year-old male who is "acting crazy." As you climb up the stairs to the third floor, you find the manager of the hotel next to the patient. The manager states that the patient was a long-time heavy drinker who had begun to attend nearby church meetings and decided 3 days ago to just stop drinking. Not seeing the patient for the past 2 days, the manager called the police to break down the door of his apartment. Upon entering the apartment, you find the patient lying in his bed, tremulous, weak, sweating, and arousable but very irritable. Your partner recorded the following set of vital signs: blood pressure 180/104, respirations 20 breaths per minute, and pulse 124 beats per minute. As you contact medical control and present the case, the telemetry physician may ask you to administer which of the following medications?

(A) IV lidocaine
(B) IV diazepam (Valium)
(C) IV diphenylhydantoin (Dilantin)
(D) IV flumazenil (Mazecon)

533. You receive a dispatch to a farm on the north side of town. As you pull up to the house, you are met by a young girl, who states that her father is out behind the house and is very sick. As you approach the patient, his wife states that her husband was working out in the fields for the past 5 hours, on an unusually hot spring day, with his shirt off. She also notes that she found a letter this afternoon, under the kitchen table, notifying farmers that all fields were going to be sprayed with insecticides by airplane today. She did not think that her husband was aware of it. About 10 minutes ago, she looked out her kitchen window and saw her husband staggering out of the fields and then suddenly collapsing. As you begin to examine this 40-year-old, muscular man, you notice that he appears unconscious, with tearing eyes and profuse salivation. He has been vomiting and has been incontinent of urine and diarrhea. The patient's vital signs are blood pressure 102/68, pulse 108 beats per minute, and respirations 28 breaths per minute. He is gurgling and has constricted pupils. As you begin to establish an airway, your partner contacts medical control. All of the following are appropriate telemetry physician requests to assist you with the care of this patient EXCEPT

(A) Suction vigorously.
(B) Perform endotracheal intubation if you cannot ventilate adequately.
(C) Remove all of the patient's clothes and immediately wash him off with copious amounts of soap and water.
(D) Administer 0.5 mg IV atropine.

534. You arrive at the home of a 35-year-old female who states that she must have eaten something bad because, after going out to eat with her boyfriend about 3 to 4 hours ago, she has felt sicker and sicker. She noticed that she began to have stomach cramps about 2 hours ago and then began to have some vomiting and severe diarrhea, which has not abated. Her vital signs are as follows: blood pressure 112/74 supine and 88/62 sitting up, pulse 94 beats per minute supine and 132 beats per minute sitting up, and respirations 18 breaths per minute. On the basis of this presentation, all of the following would be appropriate parts of the Paramedic's emergency care EXCEPT

(A) endotracheal intubation
(B) IV fluids
(C) obtaining samples of any contaminated food brought home
(D) high-flow oxygen

TOXICOLOGY

A N S W E R S

511. The answer is D. (Brady, *Toxicology and Substance Abuse*.) (A), (B), (C), and injection are the four routes of exposure for toxicologic emergencies. (D) is incorrect because aspiration occurs when a patient vomits or regurgitates the stomach contents and it passes into the respiratory tract. This often results in pneumonia. However, this is not a toxicologic route of exposure.

512. The answer is C. (Mosby, *Toxicology, Drug Abuse, and Alcoholism*.) (A), (B), and (D) are correct. (C) is incorrect because the regional poison centers act in a consultative manner to everyone involved in toxicologic emergencies but routinely do not provide on-site care to the patient.

513. The answer is D. (Caroline/Little Brown, *Poisons, Drugs, and Alcohol*.) (D) is correct.

514. The answer is D. (Caroline/Little Brown, *Poisons, Drugs, and Alcohol*.) (D) is correct. This tells us that a high percentage of poisonings are preventable.

515. The answer is B. (Caroline/Little Brown, *Poisons, Drugs, and Alcohol*.) (A), (C), (D), a patient with a myocardial infarction, and a patient with certain categories of poisonings, such as corrosives, hydrocarbons, iodides, silver nitrate, and strychnine, are all contraindications to inducing vomiting. If unsure, it is important to call your regional poison control center and/or medical control to discuss the issue. (B) is incorrect because acetaminophen (Tylenol) poisoning is not a contraindication to inducing vomiting.

516. The answer is B. (Caroline/Little Brown, *Poisons, Drugs, and Alcohol*.) (A), (C), and (D) are all correct options. (B) is incorrect because colon lavage is not part of a treatment regimen for any toxicologic emergency.

517. The answer is C. (Caroline/Little Brown, *Poisons, Drugs, and Alcohol.*) (C) is correct because caustic ingestions can produce soft-tissue damage to the larynx, epiglottis, and/or vocal cords, which may result in upper airway obstruction. (A) and (B) are incorrect in caustic ingestions because, in the process of vomiting, the actual ingested material may produce additional airway and esophageal injury and aspiration. (D) is incorrect because trying to neutralize an alkali ingestion, such as Drano lye, by giving a mild acid generates heat and may produce a thermal injury as well.

518. The answer is D. (Mosby, *Toxicology, Drug Abuse, and Alcoholism*; Mosby/ACEP, *Poisoning and Overdose.*) (D) is correct because this child with a hydrocarbon ingestion is demonstrating respiratory distress or failure and requires aggressive airway and breathing management. With hydrocarbon ingestions, the child often aspirates the substance into the lungs. This can result in respiratory distress due to noncardiogenic pulmonary edema. (A) is incorrect because the child needs more aggressive airway and breathing management. (B) is incorrect because routinely you do not want to risk the chance that the vomiting may increase aspiration into the lungs. However, sometimes the poison control consultant may recommend syrup of ipecac if the ingested substance contains a large amount of another toxin. If stomach emptying is recommended, then inducing vomiting is felt to have less risk of aspiration than performing gastric lavage. (C) is incorrect because this is non-cardiogenic pulmonary edema, and morphine would not be beneficial and even may be harmful by causing respiratory depression.

519. The answer is A. (Caroline/Little Brown, *Poisons, Drugs, and Alcohol.*) (B), (C), and (D) are correct. (A) is incorrect because, while carbon monoxide causes the most accidental and suicidal deaths from poisoning in the United States each year, it is not a part of each inhalation poisoning.

520. The answer is D. (Mosby, *Toxicology, Drug Abuse, and Alcoholism.*) (A), (B), (C), methane, ammonia, inert gases, propane, and various hydrocarbons are all causes of inhalation poisoning. (D) is incorrect because aspirin is a common form of poisoning by ingestion.

521. The answer is D. (Brady, *Toxicology and Substance Abuse.*) (A), (B), (C), and performing primary and secondary assessments are all parts of the emergency care of the carbon monoxide–poisoned patient. (D) is incorrect because you should never enter the toxic environment without respiratory protective breathing apparatus.

522. The answer is B. (Caroline/Little Brown, *Poisons, Drugs, and Alcohol.*) (A), (C), (D), and drunken behavior that resolves rapidly are all possible signs of inhalant abuse. (B) is incorrect and unrelated to an inhaled poison.

523. The answer is A. (Caroline/Little Brown, *Poisons, Drugs, and Alcohol.*) (B), (C), (D), hornet, yellow jacket, ant, scorpion, and snakebites are all examples of injected poisoning. (A) is incorrect because a dog bite may result in an infection or possibly rabies but not usually in poisoning.

524. **The answer is D.** (Caroline/Little Brown, *Poisons, Drugs, and Alcohol.*) (D) is the correct method for removal of the stinger. (A) and (B) are both incorrect because squeezing of the stinger will only pump more of the venom into the wound. (C) is simply incorrect.

525. **The answer is D.** (Brady, *Toxicology and Substance Abuse.*) (A), (B), (C), nausea, vomiting, sweating, seizures, paralysis, hypertension, diminished level of consciousness, and severe back, chest, or shoulder pain with an upper-extremity bite are all possible physical findings. (D) is incorrect because it is unrelated to a black widow spider bite.

526. **The answer is D.** (Brady, *Toxicology and Substance Abuse.*) (D) is correct because it encompasses poisoning from all possible drugs. (A) is incorrect because taking prescription drugs too rapidly may or may not cause side effects, but usually not toxic effects. (B) is incorrect because drug overdose pertains to poisoning from legal or illegal drugs. (C) is incorrect because, while many overdoses are combinations of alcohol and other drugs, it usually does not occur with normal doses of prescribed medications.

527. **The answer is D.** (Mosby/ACEP, *Drugs of Abuse.*) (A), (B), and (C) are all part of the care of this unresponsive, respiratorily depressed, alcohol- (and possible other substances) overdosed patient. (D) is incorrect because you never want to induce vomiting in a patient with a decreased level of consciousness, particularly in a patient without a gag reflex, for fear of aspiration.

528. **The answer is B.** (Mosby/ACEP, *Drugs of Abuse.*) Since barbiturate overdoses are basically treated with supportive treatment, (A), (C), (D), ventilatory support if needed, and dopamine if needed are possible parts of the emergency care. (B) is incorrect because, even though the patient has a positive gag reflex, she still has a decreased level of consciousness, with the potential to become much worse, if she truly took 90 phenobarbital (30-mg) tablets.

529. **The answer is D.** (Mosby/ACEP, *Drugs of Abuse.*) (A), (B), and (C) are correct for these common complications of a cocaine overdose. (D) is incorrect because, even though flumazenil (Mazecon) is truly the antidote for benzodiazepine overdoses, such as with diazepam (Valium), it should not be given to a patient with a cocaine overdose. The flumazenil antidote would eliminate the benefits of the benzodiazepines in controlling seizures and in calming the patient.

530. **The answer is A.** (Brady, *Toxicology and Substance Abuse.*) (B), (C), and (D) are all correct. (A) is incorrect because, while a cocaine overdose patient may be euphoric and have dilated pupils, he or she usually has tachycardic heart rhythms, such as sinus tachycardia, supraventricular tachycardia, or even ventricular tachycardia, but usually not bradyarrhythmias.

531. Answers. (Mosby/ACEP, *Drugs of Abuse.*)

    (A) 5

    (B) 7

    (C) 2

    (D) 4

    (E) 8

    (F) 3

    (G) 6

    (H) 1

532. The answer is B. (Brady, *Toxicology and Substance Abuse.*) Since this patient's presentation is most consistent with alcohol withdrawal, the medical control physician may request that you administer IV diazepam (Valium), which may be repeated initially on a 1- to 2-hour basis. The Valium would be administered in order to prevent seizures from delirium tremens (the DTs), which has a significant mortality rate. (A), (C), and (D) are incorrect because they are not the first-line medication administered for alcohol withdrawal.

533. The answer is D. (Brady, *Toxicology and Substance Abuse.*) (A), (B), and (C) are all possible appropriate recommendations from the telemetry physician for a patient presenting with organophosphate poisoning from insecticide spray. (D) is incorrect because, although atropine is actually an antidote for organophosphate poisoning, the dosage in adults is 2 to 5 mg IV every 10 to 15 minutes until the secretions are drying up.

534. The answer is A. (Brady, *Toxicology and Substance Abuse.*) (B), (C), and (D) are correct parts of the emergency care rendered by the Paramedic to the patient suffering food poisoning. (A) is incorrect because, while some types of food poisoning, such as paralytic shellfish poisoning, may result in respiratory distress or arrest, this is clearly not the case in this patient.

HEMATOLOGY

Directions: Each item below contains four suggested responses. Select the **one best** response to each item.

535. All of the following are parts of the hematopoietic (blood cell–producing) system EXCEPT

(A) liver
(B) red bone marrow
(C) yellow bone marrow
(D) spleen

536. All of the following are correct statements concerning red blood cells (RBCs) EXCEPT

(A) RBCs are the most abundant blood cells and are responsible for tissue oxygenation.
(B) Myoglobin is the key molecule in RBCs, which enables the blood to efficiently transport oxygen.
(C) When RBCs become old or damaged, they are removed from the blood by the spleen.
(D) RBC production is increased in response to anemia, hypoxia, high altitudes, or pulmonary disease.

537. All of the following are true statements about anemia EXCEPT

(A) In the adult, the most common cause of anemia is abnormal RBC production.
(B) Anemia is defined as a reduction in the level of circulating RBCs.
(C) Some symptoms of anemia include weakness, fatigue, headache, tiredness, and syncope.
(D) Some physical findings of anemia are tachypnea, tachycardia, and orthostatic hypotension.

538. You are dispatched to the home of a 41-year-old female for weakness and difficulty breathing. As you enter the patient's living room, you see that the patient is lying on the couch and appears very weak. She states that she has been told of being anemic due to very heavy menstrual periods due to uterine fibroids. She is a single parent of three small children and has been unable to find the time to have the fibroids removed, as recommended by her gynecologist. Her vital signs are blood pressure 104/68 supine and 60 palpable sitting up, pulse 110 beats per minute supine and 148 beats per minute sitting up, and respiration 28 breaths per minute. All of the following are parts of the prehospital emergency care for suspected anemia EXCEPT

(A) nasal oxygen 2 to 3 liters/minute
(B) IV fluids
(C) ECG monitoring
(D) frequently repeated measurement of vital signs

539. All of the following are correct statements about white blood cells (WBCs) EXCEPT

(A) WBCs are part of the body's immunological system, which defends against infection.
(B) WBCs are produced in the red bone marrow in adults and are destroyed in the spleen.
(C) WBCs act in the spleen and are transported by the bone marrow.
(D) Measurement of the WBC count is helpful in determining the presence of infection or disease.

540. All of the following are leukocyte (WBC) disorders EXCEPT

(A) acute leukemia
(B) chronic leukemia
(C) leukopenia
(D) anemia

541. You are sent to a 21-year-old African-American male who is complaining of "pain all over." As you enter the patient's home and begin to take a history, the patient tells you that he has sickle cell anemia. He usually has one or two attacks per year. Two days ago, he developed a cold with sneezing, a cough, and generalized achiness. However, last night he began to feel severe pain in his arms and legs, both sides of his chest, and his abdomen. He took some Advil and Tylenol, with no relief. He also complains of feeling a little short of breath. The patient's vital signs are blood pressure 130/80, pulse 100 beats per minute, and respiration 24 breaths per minute. On physical examination, the patient appears to be uncomfortable and in pain, and has a few rhonchi and no rales on lung examination. The heart examination reveals a heart rate of 110 beats per minute. The abdominal examination shows active bowel sounds, and the abdomen is soft and diffusely tender. The extremities all demonstrate muscular tenderness and are without edema or cyanosis. The prehospital emergency medical care by a Paramedic includes all of the following EXCEPT

(A) high-concentration oxygen with a nonrebreather mask
(B) IV fluids
(C) morphine sulfate 2 to 3 mg IV
(D) rapid transport

542. You are dispatched to a dentist's office for a 12-year-old boy with persistent, heavy bleeding after a routine tooth extraction. As you enter the dentist's office, you immediately are escorted to the patient, in the dentist's chair, with the dentist applying direct pressure to the bleeding site in the boy's mouth. The dentist states that he had no difficulty extracting the tooth, but he cannot stop the bleeding. As you begin to approach the patient, his mother tells you that the patient had a minor injury to his left knee about 2 months ago and had a large amount of bleeding into the joint. Since then, an occasional squeeze of his arm results in bruising. He also had a spontaneous nosebleed one night last week. He does not take any medications. His vital signs are blood pressure 102/78 lying down and 88 systolic sitting up, pulse 100 beats per minute lying down and 128 beats per minute sitting up, and respiration of 18 breaths per minute. All of the following are possible causes of this patient's bleeding episodes EXCEPT

(A) warfarin (Coumadin) overdose
(B) acute leukemia
(C) anemia
(D) hemophilia

543. All of the following are correct statements about platelets EXCEPT

(A) They are essential for blood coagulation and control of bleeding.
(B) Like RBCs and WBCs, they are the third line of cells in the blood.
(C) They live about 10 days.
(D) They are produced in the bone marrow and are removed from the circulation in the spleen.

HEMATOLOGY

A N S W E R S

535. The answer is C. (Mosby/ACEP, *Principles of Pathophysiology.*) (A), (B), and (D) are correct. (C) is incorrect because, in the fetus, blood cell production occurs in the liver (A) and the spleen (D). After birth, the red bone marrow (B) takes over the production. As the body matures, some of the red bone marrow becomes replaced by fat. This is known as the yellow bone marrow, which is inactive.

536. The answer is B. (Mosby/ACEP, *Principles of Pathophysiology.*) (A), (C), and (D) are correct. (B) is incorrect because hemoglobin, not myoglobin, is the key molecule in RBCs and is responsible for the blood's efficient transport of oxygen.

537. The answer is A. (Mosby/ACEP, *Conditions by Diagnosis.*) (B), (C), and (D) are correct. (A) is incorrect because, in the adult, chronic blood loss is the most common cause of anemia.

538. The answer is A. (Mosby/ACEP, *Conditions by Diagnosis.*) (B), (C), and (D) are correct. (A) is incorrect because a patient with suspected anemia, particularly one with orthostatic signs, should be treated with high-concentration oxygen by nonrebreather mask.

539. The answer is C. (Mosby/ACEP, *Principles of Pathophysiology.*) (A), (B), and (D) are correct. (C) is incorrect because WBCs act in the tissues and are transported by the blood.

540. The answer is D. (Mosby/ACEP, *Conditions by Diagnosis.*) (A), (B), and (C) are correct. (D) is incorrect because anemia is an RBC disorder.

541. The answer is C. (Mosby/ACEP, *Conditions by Diagnosis.*) (A), (B), and (D) are correct. (C) is incorrect even though, at the hospital, a patient having a sickle cell crisis will be treated with narcotics. However, it is essential that the patient's chest, abdominal, and extremity pain be evaluated in the emergency department prior to the administration of narcotics in order to rapidly diagnoses and properly treat emergent conditions, such as acute appendicitis, pneumothorax, and so on.

542. **The answer is C.** (Mosby/ACEP, *Conditions by Diagnosis.*) (A), (B), and (D) are all correct possibilities. Warfarin (Coumadin) is an anticoagulant, which can result in severe bleeding if too much is taken. (B) Acute leukemia is a disease characterized by abnormal increases in the number and immaturity of WBCs, which interfere with the production of platelets and can cause bleeding. (D) Hemophilia is a hereditary disease caused by a lack of one or more factors necessary for coagulation of the blood. This case presentation is most typical of a patient suffering from hemophilia. (C) is incorrect because bleeding causes anemia, not vice versa.

543. **The answer is B.** (Mosby/ACEP, *Principles of Pathophysiology.*) (A), (C), and (D) are correct. (B) is incorrect because platelets are disk-shaped fragments and are not cells.

ENVIRONMENTAL EMERGENCIES

Directions: Each item below contains four suggested responses. Select the **one best** response to each item.

544. Which of the following is the best definition of an environmental emergency?

(A) an emergency occurring to another person who is physically near to you

(B) a medical emergency related to environmental conditions

(C) a patient's garden and/or lawn being dried up from the summer heat

(D) a medical emergency occurring in a foreign country

545. All of the following are environmental factors that may affect the care of an emergently ill patient EXCEPT

(A) alcohol

(B) heat

(C) ionizing radiation

(D) cold

546. All of the following are mechanisms the body uses to eliminate heat EXCEPT

(A) vasoconstriction

(B) increased respiratory rate

(C) perspiration

(D) increased cardiac output

547. You arrive at the apartment of a 90-year-old female in the middle of a hot summer day. As you enter, you notice that it is feels very hot, all of the windows are closed, and the patient is lying on the bed dressed with a sweater and winter coat. As you begin to examine the patient, you notice that her skin is hot and dry and she is very confused and disoriented as to place and time. Her vital signs are blood pressure 70 systolic, a regular pulse of 140 beats per minute, and shallow respirations at a rate of 42 breaths per minute. As you begin to remove her clothing, the patient begins to have a generalized seizure. Which of the following best describes this patient's condition?

(A) heat stroke
(B) heat cramps
(C) heat exhaustion
(D) viral flu syndrome

548. All of the following are parts of the prehospital emergency care of the patient suffering from heat stroke EXCEPT

(A) rapid cooling of the patient using ice water–soaked sheets, ice packs, and fans
(B) nasal oxygen at 2 to 3 liters/minute
(C) rapid administration of IV fluids
(D) ECG monitoring

549. All of the following are correct statements concerning body temperatures EXCEPT

(A) Heat stroke is usually associated with a temperature of at least 105°F.
(B) Mild hypothermia is associated with a temperature between 94 and 97°F.
(C) Severe hypothermia is associated with a temperature less than 86°F.
(D) Lethal hypothermia is associated with a temperature of less than 80°F.

550. Which of the following is a correct definition of hypothermia?

(A) a clinically dead person with a pulse
(B) a generalized cooling of the body due to exposure to low temperatures
(C) a condition in which a patient is shivering
(D) a clinical state occurring only during the snow season

551. On a freezing winter's night, you are dispatched to a park for a 68-year-old male reported to be cold and confused. As you approach the patient, you notice that he is shivering, confused, and ambulating with a stumbling gait. Which of the following is the best categorization of this patient's condition?

(A) mild to moderate hypothermia
(B) severe hypothermia
(C) frostbite
(D) alcohol intoxication

552. Which of the following is the best definition of frostbite?

(A) a bitelike injury occurring in frosty snow

(B) a rare insect bite occurring in frosty snow

(C) a localized injury due to freezing of body tissues

(D) hypothermia induced by prolonged exposure to frosty snow

553. Which of the following is the best explanation of the difference between superficial and deep frostbite?

(A) Superficial frostbite produces only pale skin, while deep frostbite produces black skin.

(B) In superficial frostbite, after several days, blackened tissue peels away, revealing shiny, red skin beneath, while in deep frostbite eventually black eschar mummifies and sloughs away from viable tissue.

(C) In superficial frostbite, rewarming is painless, with blisters forming within 24 hours, while in deep frostbite blisters never form.

(D) Superficial frostbite initially is painless, while in deep frostbite the tissue becomes pink and warm after rewarming.

554. All of the following are parts of the emergency care of a patient with frostbite EXCEPT

(A) elevation and protection of the involved extremity

(B) vigorous rubbing of the involved extremity

(C) not allowing the patient to walk if the patient's lower extremity is affected by frostbite

(D) rapid transport to the hospital

555. Near-drowning is best defined as

(A) Death occurs within 24 hours of submersion.

(B) The patient suffers submersion near another patient who has just drowned.

(C) The patient suffers submersion and becomes depressed from a nearby drowning.

(D) The patient suffers submersion, but death either does not occur or occurs in more than 24 hours.

556. While in a "wet" drowning patient a significant amount of water enters the lungs, in a "dry" drowning patient a significant amount of water does not enter the lungs, because of

(A) hot, humid weather

(B) drowning in very shallow water

(C) the patient's actually dying of respiratory arrest prior to falling into the water and then drowning

(D) laryngospasm

557. You are dispatched to the town beach for a man drowning. As you drive up to the ocean, you find a 48-year-old man lying on the wet sand, with the lifeguards performing two-person CPR. The patient's wife stated that he appeared to be taken out by the undertow. All of the following are parts of the emergency care of the near-drowning patient EXCEPT

(A) If there is any possibility of a neck injury, maintain the neck in a neutral position on a wooden backboard.

(B) Since the airway is obstructed by water, administer the Heimlich maneuver.

(C) Perform endotracheal intubation and ventilate with 100 percent oxygen.

(D) If possible, try to administer positive end-expiratory pressure to keep the alveoli from collapsing.

558. Which of the following is the best definition of scuba diving?

(A) self-confined usable breathing abnormality

(B) sudden-contained underwater breathing access

(C) sorted containable unused breathing airway

(D) self-contained underwater breathing apparatus

559. You are dispatched to a summer cabin for a 24-year-old man who had been scuba diving in the local springs about 2 hours ago. Since arriving back at the cabin, he has complained of itchy skin, joint aches, diffuse numbness, and weakness of all of his extremities. When the patient began to stagger and actually fell, his roommates called 911. As you begin to assess the patient, you find the following vital signs: blood pressure 120/70, respiration 18 breaths per minute, and a regular pulse of 90 beats per minute. On examination, the patient is now found to be paraplegic. Which of the following is the best explanation for this patient's problems?

(A) air embolism

(B) acute cerebrovascular accident

(C) decompression sickness

(D) seizure disorder

560. Which of the following is the most important part of the emergency care for a patient with decompression sickness?

(A) transportation to a hyperbaric center

(B) administration of 100 percent oxygen with positive end-expiratory pressure

(C) IV fluids

(D) IV naloxone (Narcan)

561. You are assigned to a "sick diver" at a local ocean beach. The patient was diving several miles out in the ocean for over an hour. Upon resurfacing, the patient immediately complained to friends of a rapid onset of an acute tearing chest pain accompanied by right-sided paralysis. The patient was driven quickly by motorboat to the shore. As you approach the patient, you note that he is weak, confused, tachypneic, and not moving his right upper and lower extremities. The patient's vital signs are blood pressure 158/52, pulse 114 beats per minute, and a respiratory rate of 32 breaths per minute. All of the following are parts of the emergency care of this patient EXCEPT

(A) Administer 100 percent oxygen by nonrebreather mask.
(B) Sit upright on the stretcher.
(C) Monitor vital signs frequently.
(D) Transport to a hyperbaric center.

562. Which of the following is the best definition of high-altitude sickness?

(A) On exposure to reduced atmospheric pressures, hypobaric hypoxia occurs.
(B) Upon walking up a mountain, the patient becomes anxious.
(C) Upon flying in an airplane, upon assent, the patient feels his or her ears pop.
(D) On exposure to reduced atmospheric pressures, the patient begins to feel nervous.

563. All of the following are true statements concerning acute mountain sickness EXCEPT

(A) It usually occurs after rapid ascent to elevations of 5000 feet.
(B) Symptoms occur because of decreased oxygen saturation in the blood.
(C) Symptoms may include headache, dizziness, nausea, vomiting, and irritability.
(D) The most important part of the treatment is descent to a lower altitude.

564. You are dispatched to a ski lodge for a 40-year-old man with difficulty breathing. As you arrive at the patient's bedside, you are told that the patient had taken a hike up to the top of a nearby mountain 2 days ago and was in the middle of carrying all of his family's skiing equipment and suitcases into the car when he acutely complained of difficulty breathing. The patient's family note that he has never been sick before and has been in excellent health. As you approach the patient, you note that he is extremely short of breath, cyanotic, and coughing up pink frothy sputum. His vital signs reveal a blood pressure of 174/102, a pulse of 124 beats per minute, and a respiratory rate of 42 breaths per minute. The patient is very lethargic and confused. On listening to the patient's chest, you note that he has diffuse crackles. All of the following are parts of the emergency care of this patient EXCEPT

(A) 100 percent oxygen by non-rebreather
(B) stabilization before any transport is undertaken
(C) oral or intramuscular dexamethasone (Decadron) every 6 hours
(D) avoiding IV furosemide and morphine

565. All of the following are correct statements concerning high-altitude cerebral edema EXCEPT

(A) There is progression of global cerebral symptoms of acute mountain sickness.
(B) It is probably caused by increased intracranial pressure.
(C) Immediate oxygen is the most important part of the treatment.
(D) The patient may progress to stupor and coma.

ENVIRONMENTAL EMERGENCIES

A N S W E R S

544. The answer is B. (Brady, *Environmental Emergencies.*) (B) is correct. Being able to recognize them promptly and understanding their causes can lead to your rapid treatment of these various conditions. (A), (C), and (D) are incorrect.

545. The answer is A. (Brady, *Environmental Emergencies.*) (B), (C), (D), and pressure disorders are some environmental factors that may affect care. (A) is incorrect because it is not an environmental factor, even though it certainly could have an affect on the care.

546. The answer is A. (Brady, *Environmental Emergencies.*) (B), (C), (D), a decrease in heat production, and vasodilation are mechanisms. (A) is incorrect because vasoconstriction is actually one of the body's mechanisms to conserve heat.

547. The answer is A. (Caroline/Little Brown, *Environmental Emergencies.*) (A) is correct. (B) is incorrect because heat cramps present as painful cramps in the fingers, arms, legs, or abdominal muscles following strenuous activity in a hot environment. (C) is incorrect because heat exhaustion is usually seen in a patient who is working or exercising in a hot environment with a low fluid intake and has signs of dehydration: orthostatic hypotension, dizziness, syncope, headache, nausea, vomiting, diarrhea, muscle cramps, and moist cool skin. (D) is also incorrect.

548. The answer is B. (Brady, *Environmental Emergencies.*) (A), (C), (D), 100 percent oxygen, and monitoring core temperature are correct. (B) is incorrect because the patient requires 100 percent oxygen by nonrebreather mask or assisted by a bag-valve-mask if the patient's respirations are shallow.

549. The answer is D. (Brady, *Environmental Emergencies.*) (A), (B), and (C) are correct. Also, modest hypothermia is associated with a temperature between 86 and 94°F. (D) is incorrect because there is no such category as lethal hypothermia.

550. The answer is B. (Caroline/Little Brown, *Environmental Emergencies.*) (B) is correct. (A), (C), and (D) may be associated with the cold weather, but they are all incorrect.

551. The answer is A. (Brady, *Environmental Emergencies.*) (A) is correct. (B) is incorrect because patients suffering from severe hypothermia stop shivering and proceed from confusion to stupor and coma. (C) is incorrect because it represents localized injury. (D) is incorrect because, without signs of alcohol on the patient's breath and any signs of recent alcohol intake, this alone is unlikely.

552. The answer is C. (Mosby, *Environmental Emergencies.*) (C) is the best definition. (A) and (B) are incorrect because frostbite is unrelated to any kind of a bite and may occur in any freezing climate, not only frosty. (D) is incorrect because frostbite is a localized injury that may or may not be accompanied by hypothermia.

553. The answer is B. (Mosby, *Environmental Emergencies.*) (B) is correct. (A) is incorrect because superficial frostbite produces blisters, which turn into black eschar, while deep frostbite produces mottled blue or gray skin, which later forms a black eschar. (C) is incorrect because superficial frostbite rewarming is extremely painful, and, in deep frostbite, deep purple blisters may appear in 1 to 3 weeks. (D) is incorrect because in superficial frostbite the patient feels coldness and numbness, and in deep frostbite the foot remains cold, mottled, and blue or gray after rewarming.

554. The answer is B. (Mosby, *Environmental Emergencies.*) (A), (C), (D), and changing all of the patient's restrictive and wet clothing in order to prevent hypothermia are all parts of the emergency care. (B) is incorrect because vigorous rubbing is ineffective and potentially harmful. Also, partial slow rewarming with blankets is injurious.

555. The answer is D. (Brady, *Environmental Emergencies.*) (D) is correct. (A) is incorrect because usually death does not occur or occurs after 24 hours in near-drowning. (B) and (C) are incorrect because near-drowning is unrelated to being near another drowning victim.

556. The answer is D. (Mosby, *Environmental Emergencies.*) (D) is correct because, in 10 to 15 percent of drownings, a patient dies during laryngospasm, which is a part of the body's response to a very small amount of water being aspirated into the larynx. (A), (B), and (C) are all incorrect.

557. The answer is B. (Caroline/Little Brown, *Respiratory Emergencies.*) (A), (C), and (D) are correct. (B) is incorrect because performing the Heimlich maneuver in the drowning patient will not remove water from the lungs but may displace water from the stomach into the lungs.

558. **The answer is D.** (Brady, *Environmental Emergencies.*) (D) is correct. (A), (B), and (C) are incorrect.

559. **The answer is C.** (Caroline/Little Brown, *Respiratory Emergencies.*) (C) is the classic presentation of decompression sickness, initially with joint aches, known as "bends," with multiple sensory and motor abnormalities due to cerebral dysfunction, staggering gait due to cerebellar dysfunction, and finally paraplegia due to spinal cord dysfunction. (A) is incorrect because a patient suffering from an air embolism usually presents as a diver having a sudden loss of consciousness immediately upon surfacing. (B) is incorrect because, with a cerebrovascular accident, a patient would present with an acute focal neurologic weakness or paralysis. (D) is incorrect because there was no historical evidence suggesting any seizure activity.

560. **The answer is A.** (Caroline/Little Brown, *Respiratory Emergencies.*) (A) is correct, even though (B) and (C) are a part of the emergency care of the patient with decompression sickness. (B) and (C) are incorrect because they are not the most important part of the emergency care. (D) is incorrect because IV naloxone (Narcan) is not related to the care of the patient with decompression sickness.

561. **The answer is B.** (Brady, *Environmental Emergencies.*) (A), (C), (D), assessing the ABCs, and considering the administration of IV corticosteroids are correct parts of the emergency care of a patient suffering an air embolism. Also, if the patient requires air transport, it is very important to use pressurized airplanes or to fly at a low altitude. (B) is incorrect because, even though the patient is tachypneic, it is important to place the patient in the left lateral Trendelenburg position. This position keeps air bubbles away from the brain and coronary arteries.

562. **The answer is A.** (Mosby, *Environmental Emergencies.*) (A) is the correct definition. (B), (C), and (D) all may occur in the setting described but do not represent high-altitude sickness.

563. **The answer is A.** (Caroline/Little Brown, *Respiratory Emergencies*; Mosby/ACEP, *Conditions by Diagnosis.*) (B), (C), and (D) are correct. (A) is incorrect because it usually occurs after rapid ascent to elevations above 8200 feet.

564. **The answer is B.** (Caroline/Little Brown, *Respiratory Emergencies*; Mosby, *Environmental Emergencies.*) (A), (C), and (D) are all correct. (B) is incorrect because, in high-altitude pulmonary edema, the mainstay of treatment is immediate descent to a lower altitude.

565. **The answer is C.** (Mosby/ACEP, *Environmental Emergencies*; Mosby, *Environmental Emergencies.*) (A), (B), and (D) are correct. (C) is incorrect because, even though 100 percent oxygen is a very important part of the treatment of high-altitude cerebral edema, descent to a lower altitude is the most important part of the emergency care.

INFECTIOUS AND COMMUNICABLE DISEASES

Directions: Each item below contains four suggested responses. Select the **one best** response to each item.

566. All of the following are possible causes of infectious and/or communicable diseases EXCEPT

(A) bacteria
(B) parasites
(C) viruses
(D) carcinoma

567. All of the following are parts of the human body's host defense mechanism against infections EXCEPT

(A) the circulatory system
(B) the lymphatic system
(C) T lymphocytes
(D) B lymphocytes

568. All of the following are routes of exposure for the potential transmission of infectious diseases EXCEPT

(A) fecal-oral
(B) blood borne
(C) airborne
(D) talking to an exposed individual

569. All of the following are included in universal precautions EXCEPT

(A) immediate vaccinations
(B) wearing gloves and other barrier precautions
(C) hand washing
(D) use of sharp containers to discard needles, syringes, scalpels, sponges, and the like

570. HIV infection may be transmitted by all of the following body secretions EXCEPT

(A) blood
(B) vaginal secretions
(C) semen
(D) feces

571. You arrive at the apartment of a 41-year-old male with AIDS who is complaining of fever, chills, and shortness of breath with any activity. He admits to previously being diagnosed with hepatitis B, amebiasis, and Kaposi's sarcoma of the skin. All of the following are parts of the universal precautions, which need to be instituted before beginning to examine and treat this patient, EXCEPT

(A) wearing gloves
(B) carefully recapping each used needle before putting it in a sharps container
(C) placing all soiled bandages in a puncture-resistant container
(D) considering use of masks, protective eye wear, or face shields if any procedure to be performed may cause blood droplets or body fluids

572. You are dispatched to a 72-year-old male who is having fever and just feels very sick. As you arrive at the patient's home, the patient's wife tells you that he has had a high fever for 6 to 7 days, along with a productive cough, occasionally mixed with blood. The patient also complains of night sweats and a 10-lb weight loss. The wife states that her husband has been volunteering at a local hospital with patients dying from myriad illnesses and infections. Your examination reveals a blood pressure of 110/68, respirations of 22 breaths per minute, and a pulse of 110 beats per minute. The patient is hot to touch. His chest reveals a few rhonchi, and his heart rate is 100 beats per minute and regular, without any murmurs. All of the following are important precautions to be taken in treating this patient EXCEPT

(A) Wear disposable gloves.
(B) Avoid contact with the patient's sputum.
(C) Ask the patient to wear a disposable mask.
(D) Paramedics do not need to wear masks.

573. You arrive at a local grammar school and are escorted to the nurse's office. You are informed that there have been two cases of meningitis in the past week. Both of the children are still hospitalized, and one remains in a coma. The nurse states that a 6-year-old boy was taken out of class after feeling sick. The child tells you that he feels hot, has a headache, and just wants to go to sleep. The nurse also notes that the child had vomited in the toilet. All of the following need to be done before assessing this child EXCEPT

(A) putting on disposable gloves
(B) putting a disposable mask on the patient
(C) placing all linen in bags and labeling them for the protection of laundry personnel
(D) having each Paramedic put on a disposable mask

574. At 12 noon, you are dispatched to a summer camp for an animal bite. As you walk to the playground, one of the teenage counselors directs you to a 4-year-old girl. Evidently, about an hour ago, a group of five small children approached a large "cat" that was licking its paws. The patient was scratched deeply in her right arm and was bleeding and crying. Another counselor, who observed the episode, noted that the "cat" was actually a raccoon. As you approach the patient, you can see the raccoon walking around on the side of the playground slowly, with a staggering gait. All of the following are important parts of the emergency care of this patient EXCEPT

(A) Disposable gloves are not necessary in this case.
(B) Encourage the counselors to calmly remove all of the children near the raccoon.
(C) Contact local police and an animal control agency for immediate assistance.
(D) Make sure to notify the emergency department staff of the nature of the child's wound so that they can safely take care of the child and dispose of all soiled bandages.

575. Match each of the following communicable diseases with the correct medical name.

  (A) chickenpox _____
  (B) measles _____
  (C) mumps _____
  (D) German measles _____
  (E) whooping cough _____

    1. pertussis
    2. rubeola
    3. rubella
    4. varicella
    5. mumps

576. Match each of the following communicable diseases with the correct statement.

  (A) influenza _____
  (B) measles _____
  (C) rubella _____
  (D) mononucleosis _____
  (E) pertussis _____
  (F) herpes simplex type I _____
  (G) mumps _____
  (H) chickenpox _____
  (I) herpes simplex type II _____
  (J) gastroenteritis _____

    1. causes the common cold and the flu
    2. causes cold sores around the mouth and nose
    3. German measles, red rash
    4. produces vesicles on the genitalia
    5. infection of the stomach and intestines
    6. red rash first on face and then on trunk
    7. red rash first on trunk and then on extremities
    8. swelling of salivary glands and cheeks
    9. swollen glands, fever, and enlarged spleen
   10. whooping cough

577. You arrive at the home of a 5-year-old girl, whose parents state that they found her in bed this morning with a high fever, appearing sick, and with red spots all over her skin. Two weeks ago, the child slept over her cousins' house, and one of the children had become sick the next day. As you begin to examine the child, you note that she is alert and uncomfortable, with the following vital signs: blood pressure 100/68, pulse 110 beats per minute, and respiratory rate 24 breaths per minute. The patient has discrete red spots, some of them fluid filled, on her chest, stomach, and back. All of the following are appropriate steps for the Paramedic to take in order to prevent acquiring and spreading this disease EXCEPT

(A) Wear disposable gloves.
(B) Wear a face mask.
(C) Place all linens and trash in separate bags for the protection of others.
(D) Unlike major trauma, it is not necessary to call ahead and notify the emergency department of this patient's diagnosis and arrival.

578. Which of the following illnesses are prevented by the use of the MMR vaccine?

(A) measles, meningitis, and rabies
(B) measles, mumps, and rubeola
(C) measles, mumps, and rubella
(D) measles, meningitis, and rubeola

579. You are stationed at a county fair when a teenage girl runs up to tell you that her pregnant girlfriend is going into labor. As you approach the 18-year-old patient, you notice that she is crying and appears to be very upset. She has had regular contractions for several hours, but now they are much stronger and only 3 minutes apart. Her vital signs are stable, and her water breaks on the stretcher sheets. In the back of the ambulance, the patient tells you that she is very upset because she has a flare-up of genital herpes. Which of the following is the correct reason for calling ahead and notifying the emergency department of this patient's condition and arrival?

(A) to secure an isolation room for this patient
(B) so the emergency department staff can put on masks and gowns prior to this patient's arrival
(C) because women in labor with active herpes genitalis are only delivered with forceps
(D) because women in labor with active herpes genitalis are delivered by cesarean section

580. You are dispatched to a 46-year-old homeless male in an alleyway complaining of severe itching. As you approach the patient, you notice that his hair is covered with white specks and his skin actually has small, white, moving organisms. All of the following are important parts of the treatment of this patient EXCEPT

(A) wearing disposable gloves
(B) hand washing after contact with this patient
(C) bagging and labeling all linen
(D) calling ahead to the emergency department to request an isolation bed for this patient

581. You are sent to a 67-year-old male, who is "very sick." The patient states that he began to feel sick 2 days ago and complains of abdominal cramps, nausea, and vomiting. As he began to feel a little better, he developed diarrhea. He noted that he had 15 bowel movements yesterday and now over 7 today. He is becoming concerned because he is gradually becoming weaker and has no appetite. He denies any blood in the stool, present abdominal pain, or any previous gastrointestinal diseases. The patient's vital signs are blood pressure 108/70 supine and 80 systolic palpable sitting up, pulse 90 beats per minute supine and 120 beats per minute sitting up, and respirations of 18 breaths per minute. The patient appears weak and has a dry tongue and dry mucous membranes. The patient's abdomen is soft, nondistended, and nontender, with active bowel sounds and no masses. This patient's presentation is most consistent with which of the following?

(A) viral gastroenteritis with dehydration
(B) peptic ulcer disease with dehydration
(C) acute diverticulitis with dehydration
(D) acute appendicitis with dehydration

582. You arrive at the home of a 47-year-old female who says that she saw her doctor 2 weeks ago because of severe joint pains and a rash. The patient was worried because she regularly works in her garden and has frequently removed deer ticks. However, currently she complains of severe headaches, tiredness, and difficulty concentrating. The patient's vital signs are a blood pressure of 138/80, a regular pulse of 72 beats per minute, and respirations of 16 breaths per minute. Results of the patient's examination, including a neurologic assessment, are normal. However, the patient has a large, 5-cm, red, circular rash on her back, with clearing in the middle. All of the following are complications of Lyme disease EXCEPT

(A) arthritis
(B) first-degree heart block
(C) kidney stones
(D) cranial nerve paralysis

INFECTIOUS AND COMMUNICABLE DISEASES

A N S W E R S

566. The answer is D. (Brady, *Infectious Diseases.*) (A), (B), (C), fungi, protozoans, and helminths (worms) are all possible causes. (D) is incorrect because carcinoma is the medical word for cancer, which is not infectious or communicable.

567. The answer is A. (Brady, *Infectious Diseases.*) (B), (C), and (D) are parts of the human body's defense. T lymphocytes and B lymphocytes are a part of the body's immune system. The lymphatic system is a network of lymph ducts and nodes, which help to fight infections as well. (A) is incorrect because the circulatory system is a key part of the body but does not play a direct role in fighting infections.

568. The answer is D. (Brady, *Infectious Diseases.*) (A), (B), (C), and food borne are some of the potential routes. (D) is incorrect because exposure is to patients who have a communicable disease, not to someone who was only exposed to a communicable disease.

569. The answer is A. (Caroline/Little Brown, *Communicable Diseases.*) (B), (C), and (D) are included. (A) is incorrect because, even though vaccinations may prevent the acquisition of certain communicable diseases, they are not considered a part of universal precautions.

570. The answer is D. (Brady, *Infectious Diseases.*) (A), (B), (C), and cerebrospinal fluid may transmit HIV infection. HIV may be also transmitted by tears, saliva, breast milk, amniotic fluid, and urine, but such transmissions are uncommon. (D) is incorrect.

571. The answer is B. (Brady, *Infectious Diseases.*) (A), (C), and (D) are correct. (B) is incorrect because used needles should never be recapped, because of the high incidence of needle-stick injuries.

572. The answer is D. (Mosby, *Infectious Diseases*.) (A), (B), and (C) are correct. (D) is incorrect because it is essential for the Paramedics caring for this patient to wear disposable masks in order to decrease the chance of acquiring and spreading this infection. In this case, pulmonary tuberculosis and other causes of pneumonia are possible diagnoses.

573. The answer is C. (Brady, *Infectious Diseases*.) (A), (B), and (D) are very important in order to prevent the spread of a possible case of acute meningitis. Meningitis is primarily spread through airborne droplets released by coughing or sneezing. (C) is incorrect because, even though this is very important, it is performed after the patient has been taken to the hospital.

574. The answer is A. (Mosby, *Soft Tissue Injuries and Burns*.) (B), (C), (D), wearing disposable gloves, and using universal precautions are important parts of the emergency care of this child with an animal bite and possible rabies exposure. (A) is incorrect because it is essential to wear disposable gloves in order to prevent possibly acquiring and spreading the rabies virus.

575. Answers. (Brady, *Infectious Diseases*.)
(A) 4
(B) 2
(C) 5
(D) 3
(E) 1

576. Answers. (Brady, *Infectious Diseases*; Mosby/ACEP, *Infection Control*.)
(A) 1   (F) 2
(B) 6   (G) 8
(C) 3   (H) 7
(D) 9   (I) 4
(E) 10   (J) 5

577. The answer is D. (Brady, *Infectious Diseases*.) (A), (B), (C), and hand washing are all appropriate parts of the emergency care of this child with chickenpox (varicella). (D) is incorrect because it is very important to notify the emergency department of the diagnosis and arrival of this patient so that an isolation room can be designated for her. This will decrease the exposure of other patients, families, visitors, staff, and, particularly, any pregnant women to this patient.

578. The answer is C. (Mosby/ACEP, *Infection Control*.) (C) is the correct definition of the MMR vaccine. (A) is incorrect because MMR does not prevent meningitis or rabies. (B) is incorrect because measles is the same as rubeola, and the *R* stands for rubella. (D) is incorrect for the reasons previously stated.

579. **The answer is D.** (Brady, *Infectious Diseases.*) (D) is correct. (A) and (B) are incorrect because active genital herpes does not require isolation, since it is only transmitted by direct contact with the lesions. (C) is incorrect because the use of forceps is unrelated to the pregnant mother with active herpes genitalis. It is also very important, in this case, to carefully bag all of the linens and sterilize the stretcher and mattress, since the patient's water broke and the herpes simplex II virus has contaminated the amniotic fluids.

580. **The answer is D.** (Brady, *Infectious Diseases.*) (A), (B), and (C) are correct. (D) is incorrect because patients with lice do not require isolation. The staff members treating the patient only need protective gloves, gowns, and headgear.

581. **The answer is A.** (Mosby/ACEP, *Conditions by Diagnosis.*) (A) is correct because acute viral gastroenteritis usually presents as a viral infection that causes inflammation of the stomach (nausea and/or vomiting) and the intestines (diarrhea) associated with fairly normal physical examination findings. Gastroenteritis less commonly may be caused by bacteria, parasites, or other toxins. (B) is incorrect because peptic ulcer disease usually presents with severe upper abdominal pain, and sometimes with vomiting of blood, associated with significant upper abdominal tenderness (epigastric area). (C) is incorrect because acute diverticulitis usually presents with acute focal (usually lower) abdominal pain and focal tenderness. (D) is incorrect because acute appendicitis usually presents with severe abdominal pain that is initially periumbilical and then moves down to the right lower quadrant, and abdominal examination findings of a very tender right lower quadrant.

582. **The answer is C.** (Mosby, *Toxicology, Drug Abuse, and Alcoholism.*) (A), (B), and (D) are correct. (C) is incorrect because it is not associated with Lyme disease.

BEHAVIORAL AND PSYCHIATRIC DISORDERS

Directions: Each item below contains four suggested responses. Select the **one best** response to each item.

583. Which of the following is the best definition of a psychiatric or behavioral emergency?

  (A) The patient presents with strange attire and verbalizes concerns with the country's political direction.

  (B) The patient's family calls because the patient has been verbally argumentative for the past several years.

  (C) The patient presents with a disorder of mood, thought, or behavior that is dangerous to him- or herself or to others.

  (D) The patient has been crying on and off after a spouse died from cancer 3 weeks ago.

584. Match the following terms with the correct definition or description.

  (A) affect _____
  (B) depression _____
  (C) posture _____
  (D) anxiety _____
  (E) mental status _____
  (F) anger _____

  1. sad expression, crying, and apathetic behavior
  2. sometimes caused by feelings of helplessness
  3. dominant mood of fear and apprehension
  4. means of establishing mental vital signs
  5. outward expression of a person's mood
  6. sitting at the edge of a chair or gripping the armrest

585. You are dispatched to the home of a 57-year-old hostile male who is acting "crazy." As you enter the patient's apartment, you notice the patient sitting on a kitchen chair with his arms tightly crossed and appearing very angry. As you slowly approach the patient, you notice that his friends are actually raising their voices with the patient. Which of the following is one of the best reasons for having friends, relatives, or bystanders removed from the scene of a psychiatric or behavioral emergency?

(A) They are supportive and quiet.
(B) You want to quickly restrain the patient because your shift is almost over.
(C) They truly appear to be making the situation worse and escalating any violence.
(D) You personally do not like their answers to your questions.

586. All of the following are useful interviewing skills in managing the emotionally disturbed patient EXCEPT

(A) listening to the patient in a concerned and receptive manner
(B) admonishing the patient for demonstrating any feelings
(C) providing information about aspects of the upcoming treatment at the hospital
(D) offering realistic reassurance and support

587. Which of the following is the best category for situations in which a Paramedic would be expected to transport a patient forcibly against his or her will?

(A) when the patient appears to be a danger to him- or herself or others
(B) an anxiety reaction with panic attacks
(C) a grieving widow with a number of friends present
(D) a troubled senior citizen worried about the country's future

588. All of the following are methods of restraint that may be necessary in managing an emotionally disturbed patient EXCEPT

(A) verbal restraint
(B) leather restraints
(C) mouth-gagging devices
(D) small towels, cravats, and roll bandages

589. All of the following are risk factors for suicide EXCEPT

(A) female sex, age under 40
(B) previous suicide attempt
(C) depressed or sudden improvement in depression
(D) financial setback or job loss

590. You are dispatched to a 26-year-old emotionally disturbed male. As you arrive at the patient's home, the patient is lying on the couch. The patient appears withdrawn and states that he feels "useless" after just being let go from his job. He admits to having thoughts of killing himself and even goes on to describe his plan to go to a nearby, quiet subway station and jump in front of a train. Which of the following is the correct approach to this patient?

(A) Calmly talk with the patient and encourage him to see a psychiatrist in the morning.

(B) Call medical control and request permission to administer 10 mg IV diazepam (Valium) in order to sedate the patient.

(C) Calmly interview the patient and encourage him to be transported to the hospital in order to be evaluated and treated.

(D) Leave the patient alone, proceed down to the ambulance, and call medical control to discuss the case.

BEHAVIORAL AND PSYCHIATRIC DISORDERS

ANSWERS

583. **The answer is C.** (Caroline/Little Brown, *Behavioral Emergencies.*) (C) is correct, with the key point being that the patient's behavior appears to be dangerous to him- or herself or to others. (A), (B), and (D) are incorrect because, even though the behavior may be different from that to which we are accustomed, it does not contain the elements of a psychiatric or behavioral emergency.

584. **Answers.** (Caroline/Little Brown, *Behavioral Emergencies.*)
   (A) 5
   (B) 1
   (C) 6
   (D) 3
   (E) 4
   (F) 2

585. **The answer is C.** (Caroline/Little Brown, *Behavioral Emergencies.*) (C) is correct. (A), (B), and (D) are all incorrect reasons for asking to have anyone removed from the scene of an emotionally disturbed patient.

586. **The answer is B.** (Mosby, *Behavioral Emergencies.*) (A), (C), (D), asking effective questions, and correcting cognitive misconceptions or distortions are some of the useful interviewing techniques. (B) is incorrect because the patient should be encouraged to express his or her feelings.

587. **The answer is A.** (Caroline/Little Brown, *Behavioral Emergencies.*) (A) is correct. At the hospital, if the psychiatrist has the same impression, he or she may hospitalize the patient against his or her will for a limited period of time. (B), (C), and (D) are incorrect because, even though you may be called upon to evaluate similar patients, you would be expected to transport the patient against his or her will only if the patient appeared to be a danger to him- or herself or others.

588. **The answer is C.** (Mosby, *Behavioral Emergencies and Crisis Intervention*; Caroline/ Little Brown, *Behavioral Emergencies*.) (A), (B), and (D) are some of the more common techniques used to restrain the emotionally disturbed patient. (C) is incorrect because mouth gagging is not a restraint technique and is potentially very dangerous to the patient.

589. **The answer is A.** (Caroline/Little Brown, *Behavioral Emergencies*.) (B); (C); (D); expressing suicidal thoughts and concrete suicide plans; being single, widowed, or divorced; social isolation; alcohol or drug abuse; recent loss of spouse or significant relationship; chronic debilitating illness; and family history of suicide and schizophrenia are all risk factors for suicide. (A) is incorrect because being a male over 55 years of age is a risk factor for suicide.

590. **The answer is C.** (Brady, *Behavioral and Psychiatric Emergencies*.) (C) is correct. (A) is incorrect because you should never leave a possibly suicidal patient at home. (B) is incorrect because the patient does not appear to be agitated or need to be forcibly restrained. (D) is incorrect because you should never leave this possibly suicidal patient alone, for fear that he may harm himself.

GYNECOLOGIC EMERGENCIES

Directions: Each item below contains four suggested responses. Select the **one best** response to each item.

591. Match the following female reproductive organs with the correct function.

(A) ovaries _____
(B) fallopian tubes _____
(C) uterus _____
(D) cervix _____
(E) endometrium _____
(F) vagina _____
(G) labia _____
(H) urethra _____

1. two sets of organs that protect the vagina and urethra
2. produces a menstrual period by its monthly sloughing
3. produces eggs and hormones
4. organ in which a developing fetus grows
5. dilates during labor, allowing passage of the baby
6. opening of the urinary system for draining of the bladder
7. connects the uterus with the outside of the body
8. transports eggs from the ovary to the uterus

592. All of the following are common symptoms of gynecologic emergencies EXCEPT

(A) excessive vaginal bleeding
(B) pregnancy with lower abdominal pain
(C) fever and lower abdominal pain
(D) dysuria and increased urinary frequency

593. You are dispatched to a 44-year-old female who called because of excess vaginal bleeding and extreme weakness. As you arrive at the patient's bedside, you note that there is a large amount of blood on the bed sheets. As you begin to interview the patient, she notes that she has a long-standing history of "fibroids." However, in the past few months, she has been having increasingly heavy vaginal bleeding with her periods and even in between. On physical examination, you note the following vital signs: blood pressure 96/64 supine and 60 palpable systolic sitting up, pulse 110 beats per minute supine and 140 beats per minute sitting up, and respirations 18 breaths per minute. All of the following are part of the emergency care of the patient with a gynecologic emergency EXCEPT

(A) keeping the patient supine
(B) administering oxygen and IV fluids
(C) monitoring ECG and repeat vital signs
(D) remaining on the scene and contacting medical control for additional options for stabilization at the scene

594. You arrive at one of the local college's dormitories to evaluate a 20-year-old female who is complaining of abdominal pain. As you approach the patient, she admits to having had left lower quadrant abdominal pain for the past 24 hours. She hesitantly adds that she missed her last menstrual period 3 weeks ago and has noticed some slight vaginal bleeding with the onset of the pain. She does admit to being sexually active with her boyfriend and rarely without birth control protection. On examination, the patient's vital signs are blood pressure 104/72 supine and 84 palpable systolic sitting up, pulse 96 beats per minute supine and 132 beats per minute sitting up, and respiratory rate 18 breaths per minute. The abdominal examination reveals a very tender left lower quadrant with guarding and rebound tenderness. All of the following are possible gynecologic emergencies occurring in this patient EXCEPT

(A) ectopic pregnancy
(B) acute peptic ulcer disease
(C) ruptured ovarian cyst
(D) ruptured tubo-ovarian abcess

595. You are dispatched to a possible sexual assault victim in her apartment. As you enter the room, the patient states that she was raped 4 hours ago. She lives alone and is very upset. After establishing that the patient does not have any life-threatening traumatic injuries, you proceed to document that her vital signs are all normal. All of the following are part of the care rendered to the sexual assault victim EXCEPT

(A) psychological and emotional support
(B) allowing a female to accompany the victim to the hospital
(C) trying to question the victim about the details of the incident
(D) not allowing the patient to shower, change clothes, or douche before going to the hospital

GYNECOLOGIC EMERGENCIES

ANSWERS

591. Answers. (Brady, *Gynecological Emergencies.*)
   (A) 3
   (B) 8
   (C) 4
   (D) 5
   (E) 2
   (F) 7
   (G) 1
   (H) 6

592. The answer is D. (Caroline/Little Brown, *Gynecologic Emergencies.*) (A), (B), and (C) are common symptoms of gynecologic emergencies. (D) is incorrect because dysuria and increased urinary frequency are symptoms of a urinary tract infection.

593. The answer is D. (Caroline/Little Brown, *Gynecologic Emergencies.*) (A), (B), and (C) are parts of the emergency care rendered to patients with gynecologic emergencies. (D) is incorrect because gynecologic emergencies associated with excessive bleeding should be treated as "load and go" in order to arrive at the hospital before the development of shock. This is also done in order to be able to surgically treat the cause of the bleeding, which cannot occur in the prehospital setting.

594. The answer is B. (Caroline/Little Brown, *Gynecologic Emergencies.*) (A), (C), and (D) are all gynecologic emergencies that could present in a similar manner to this patient. The triad of abdominal pain, vaginal bleeding, and amenorrhea are most suggestive of an ectopic pregnancy. (B) is incorrect because this is a gastrointestinal disease and usually presents with epigastric or right upper quadrant pain associated with nausea, vomiting, and occasionally hematemesis.

595. The answer is C. (Brady, *Gynecologic Emergencies*.) (A), (B), (D), handling clothing as little as possible, not examining the victim's perineal area, using brown paper bags to collect blood-stained articles separately, and not allowing the victim to comb her hair or clean her fingernails are all part of the care rendered to a sexual assault victim. (C) is incorrect because this will be performed at the hospital and later by the police officers.

OBSTETRICS

Directions: Each item below contains four suggested responses. Select the **one best** response to each item.

596. All of the following are correct statements concerning pregnancy EXCEPT

(A) The first trimester is the first 90 days of pregnancy and is crucial for fetal development.

(B) At 20 weeks, the fetus has a good chance of surviving if born prematurely.

(C) In the second trimester, the fetus develops bone structure, and the uterus is palpable.

(D) In the third trimester, the uterus reaches its maximal size.

597. All of the following are important approaches to assessing the obstetric patient EXCEPT

(A) obtaining key historical information, such as the mother's previous number of pregnancies and deliveries, the length of this pregnancy, and the expected delivery date

(B) history of vaginal bleeding, vaginal discharge, and ruptured membranes

(C) evaluating routine vital signs but not orthostatic vital signs

(D) abdominal examination for gross deformity, presence of masses, distended bladder, intestinal distention, or enlarged organs

598. All of the following are predelivery emergencies EXCEPT

(A) spontaneous abortion
(B) ectopic pregnancy
(C) eclampsia
(D) breech delivery

599. You are called to see a 23-year-old female who is 32 weeks pregnant and has vaginal bleeding. Upon questioning, the patient admits to having had 12 hours of vaginal bleeding associated with acute abdominal pain. The patient's vital signs are blood pressure 124/84 supine and 80/50 sitting up, pulse 104 beats per minute supine and 134 beats per minute sitting up, and respirations 16 breaths per minute. The most likely cause of this presentation is

(A) placenta previa
(B) eclampsia
(C) postpartum hemorrhage
(D) abruptio placenta

600. All of the following are correct statements concerning the three stages of labor EXCEPT

(A) In the first stage of labor, uterine contractions begin to increase in frequency, force, and duration, in association with progressive dilation of the cervix.

(B) In the first stage of labor, the average duration of uterine contractions is 8 to 12 hours and includes the rupture of the membranes.

(C) The second stage of labor is defined as the time from the full dilation of the cervix to the delivery of the baby.

(D) The third stage of labor is defined as the time from the delivery of the baby to the termination of uterine contractions.

601. You are dispatched to the home of a 36-year-old pregnant female in labor. As you walk up the stairs, the patient's husband tells you that his wife is pregnant for the fourth time. As you enter the bedroom, the patient makes eye contact with you and starts to yell, "The baby is coming." As you glance at the patient's perineal area, you see that the baby's head is crowning. All of the following are parts of the preparation for a prehospital imminent delivery EXCEPT

(A) Position the patient in a prone position, with her legs apart.
(B) Open the sterile obstetrics kit.
(C) Place sterile towels under the mother's buttocks, on the bed between the mother's legs, on the mother's abdomen and on each leg.
(D) Wash your hands thoroughly and put on sterile gloves.

602. You are flagged down on a street corner by a teenage girl stating that her aunt is about to have her seventh child in her bedroom. As you enter the bedroom, the patient, a 32-year-old female, is beginning to push, and the baby's head is about to deliver. As you quickly put on a pair of sterile gloves, you immediately prepare to assist this mother with the delivery of her child. All of the following are parts of the emergency care to be rendered for this prehospital delivery EXCEPT

(A) Put on sterile gloves.
(B) After delivery of the head, check to make sure the cord is not looped around the neck.
(C) Suction the infant's mouth and nose for the first time only after the entire delivery is completed.
(D) As the entire body delivers, be careful to grasp and support it because the baby is very slippery.

603. You are called to a college student health service for an 18-year-old student who is about to deliver. A fellow student, who is a nurse, is trying to assist the patient in doing special breathing exercises, and you take a look at the patient's perineum. You note that the baby's head is crowning, and the patient tells you that it feels like the baby is coming. As you prepare the patient with drapes, the nurse tells you that the patient broke her water about 3 hours ago and shows you a sheet that is stained with yellow-green fluid. As you realize that the patient's amniotic fluid is meconium stained, you immediately ask your partner to prepare for all of the following EXCEPT

(A) Assemble a pediatric intubation kit.
(B) As soon as the baby's head delivers, wipe the nostrils and mouth with sterile gauze and use the bulb aspirator to suction the nose and mouth.
(C) Next use the Delee suction trap to suction the mouth gently.
(D) With the delivery of the complete baby, if you note heavy meconium staining, you should contact medical control to request permission to perform intubation and to connect a meconium aspirator and begin to suction while removing the endotracheal tube. This may need to be repeated.

604. Which of the following is the correct location for clamping the umbilical cord?

(A) about 6 to 9 inches from the infant
(B) about 6 to 9 inches from the placenta
(C) about 12 to 15 inches from the placenta
(D) about 12 to 15 inches from the baby

605. All of the following are parts of providing neonatal resuscitation EXCEPT
(A) oxygen, ideally warm and humidified
(B) chest compressions with a 3:1 ratio at a rate of 120 per minute
(C) epinephrine and naloxone by endotracheal tube if there is no IV access
(D) fluid boluses administered at 20 mL/kg

606. All of the following are abnormal deliveries for which the patient must be rapidly transported to the hospital for cesarean section delivery EXCEPT

(A) buttocks breech delivery
(B) footling breech delivery
(C) transverse-lie presentation
(D) face presentation

607. You are dispatched to a birthing center for a 37-year-old female who has just delivered her sixth child after an uneventful pregnancy. However, the nurse midwife became concerned when the patient continued to have a large amount of vaginal hemorrhaging even after delivering the placenta. As you approach the patient, you note that she appears weak and pale. The patient's vital signs are blood pressure 122/72 supine and 90 systolic palpable sitting up, pulse rate 112 beats per minute supine and 138 beats per minute sitting up, and respirations 18 breaths per minute. All of the following are parts of the emergency care of the post-partum hemorrhaging patient EXCEPT

(A) Continue gentle uterine massage.
(B) Start a large-bore IV.
(C) Add 10 units of oxytocin to the IV fluid bag and administer at 20 to 30 mL/min.
(D) Gently pack the patient's vagina with sterile dressings.

OBSTETRICS

A N S W E R S

596. The answer is B. (Caroline/Little Brown, *Obstetrics and Emergency Childbirth.*) (A), (C), and (D) are correct. (B) is incorrect because a prematurely born fetus has a good chance of surviving at 28 weeks.

597. The answer is C. (Mosby, *Obstetric and Neonatal Resuscitation.*) (A), (B), and (D) are correct. (C) is incorrect because orthostatic vital signs are very important in evaluating the obstetric patient. They are very helpful in diagnosing early bleeding or fluid loss.

598. The answer is D. (Brady, *Obstetrical Emergencies.*) (A), (B), and (C) are correct. (D) is incorrect because breech delivery is an obstetrical emergency that occurs during delivery, not in the predelivery period.

599. The answer is D. (Mosby/ACEP, *Pregnancy and Childbirth.*) (D) is correct because third-trimester vaginal bleeding associated with abdominal pain is more likely due to abruptio placenta. (A) is incorrect because placenta previa is usually painless. It is defined as the placenta's being located partially or completely in front of the cervix. (B) is incorrect because eclampsia presents as seizures associated with hypertension, edema, and protein in the urine without vaginal bleeding. (C) is incorrect because postpartum hemorrhage is vaginal bleeding that occurs after delivery, not during pregnancy.

600. The answer is D. (Mosby/ACEP, *Pregnancy and Childbirth.*) (A), (B), and (C) are correct. (D) is incorrect because the third stage of labor is from the delivery of the baby until the delivery of the placenta.

601. The answer is A. (Caroline/Little Brown, *Obstetrics and Emergency Childbirth.*) (B), (C), and (D) are correct. (A) is incorrect because you should position the mother in the supine position (on her back) with her legs apart.

602. **The answer is C.** (Mosby, *Obstetrical and Neonatal Emergencies.*) (A), (B), and (D) are correct. (C) is incorrect because, after the head has been delivered and before the next contraction, you should try to suction the baby's mouth and nose. After the completed delivery, you should clean the baby's airway with sterile gauze and repeat suctioning of the mouth and nose.

603. **The answer is D.** (Mosby, *Obstetrical and Neonatal Emergencies.*) (A), (B), and (C) are correct. (D) is incorrect because, with a baby presenting with probable meconium aspiration, you need to proceed with endotracheal intubation and suctioning immediately, without contacting medical control.

604. **The answer is A.** (Mosby, *Obstetrical and Neonatal Emergencies.*) (A) is correct. The Brady text recommends that the first clamp be 10 cm from the baby and the second clamp 15 cm. (B), (C), and (D) are incorrect.

605. **The answer is D.** (Mosby/ACEP, *The Critical Pediatric Patient.*) (A), (B), and (C) are correct. (D) is incorrect because, in neonates, the correct dose for fluid administration is 10 mL/kg. In the pediatric population, the correct dose is 20 mL/kg.

606. **The answer is A.** (Caroline/Little Brown, *Obstetrics and Emergency Childbirth*; Brady, *Obstetrical Emergencies.*) (A) is correct because, if necessary, the Paramedic may assist the mother in safely delivering a buttocks breech delivery. (B), (C), and (D) are incorrect because all must be delivered at the hospital by cesarean section.

607. **The answer is D.** (Caroline/Little Brown, *Obstetrics and Emergency Childbirth.*) (A), (B), and (C) are correct. (D) is incorrect because you should never insert packs into the vagina. If the patient is hemorrhaging from perineal tears, provide firm external pressure on the site of bleeding.

SECTION VI: SPECIAL CONSIDERATIONS

The following topics are covered in Section VI:

- Neonatology
- Pediatrics
- Geriatrics
- Abuse and Assault
- Acute Interventions for Chronic Care Patients

NEONATOLOGY

Directions: Each item below contains four suggested responses. Select the **one best** response to each item.

608. A neonate is defined as

(A) a preterm newborn child
(B) a term newborn from time of birth to 1 week old
(C) an infant up to 3 months old
(D) an infant up to 1 month old

609. You are performing a field delivery. As the bag of water breaks, you notice a greenish-colored fluid. Identifying this as meconium staining, you prepare to treat the newborn to prevent meconium aspiration. As you prepare your suction equipment, you will begin suctioning

(A) as soon as the head is delivered and before the first breath
(B) after the child is delivered but before the first breath
(C) after the child is delivered and after administering the first breath
(D) after drying, warming, and providing tactile stimulation to initiate spontaneous respiration

610. After suctioning an infant, you notice thick particulate meconium in the airway. The child has depressed vital signs and is cyanotic. Your first intervention should be

(A) Administer 100 percent oxygen via "blow by."
(B) Immediately perform endotracheal intubation and attach to suction to clear the airway of meconium.
(C) Ventilate with 100 percent oxygen via bag-valve-mask.
(D) Perform tactile stimulation to increase respiratory effort.

611. You have delivered a child in the field. At 1 minute, the child has a pink body and cyanotic extremities, a pulse rate of 140, a grimace, some flexion of the extremities, and a strong cry. What is the 1-minute Apgar score for this child?

(A) 7
(B) 8
(C) 9
(D) 10

612. A premature neonate is one who is

(A) born at less than 38 weeks' gestation OR weighing less than 2500 g
(B) born at less than 28 weeks' gestation OR weighing less than 2500 g
(C) born at less than 38 weeks' gestation AND weighing less than 2500 g
(D) born at less than 28 weeks' gestation AND weighing less than 2500 g

613. You deliver a term infant. After drying, warming, stimulating, and suctioning, your next step in the resuscitative effort, based on the inverted pyramid, should be

(A) chest compressions
(B) ventilation via bag-valve-mask
(C) administration of oxygen
(D) administration of medications

614. Some pregnancies pose a high risk, which should alert the Paramedic that special resuscitative measures may be needed after the birth of the child. All of the following are problems that may occur during pregnancy that could create a high-risk birth EXCEPT

(A) antepartum hemorrhage
(B) preeclampsia
(C) multiple pregnancy (twins)
(D) breech presentation

615. The umbilical cord contains blood vessels that the Paramedic may cannulate in order to administer medications to the neonate. How many of each vessel are in the umbilical cord, and which one would the Paramedic use to cannulate for administration of medication?

(A) two veins, one artery; vein is cannulated
(B) one artery, one vein; artery is cannulated
(C) two arteries, one vein; artery is cannulated
(D) two arteries, one vein; vein is cannulated

616. What is the volume of fluid to be administered to a neonate (infant less than 1 month old) for volume expansion due to hypovolemia?

(A) 5 mL/kg
(B) 10 mL/kg
(C) 15 mL/kg
(D) 20 mL/kg

617. The neonatal dose of naloxone is

(A) 1 mg
(B) 1 mg/kg
(C) 0.1 mg/kg
(D) 0.01 mg/kg

NEONATOLOGY

ANSWERS

608. **The answer is D.** (Brady, *Emergency Management of the Neonate.*) The neonate is best described as (D), an infant less than one month of age. (A), (B), and (C) are incorrect.

609. **The answer is A.** (Mosby, *OB/GYN and Neonatal.*) (A) When meconium staining is present, the Paramedic should suction the infant's airway as soon as the head is delivered and before the shoulders are delivered. The Paramedic should be reasonably sure that all meconium has been suctioned prior to the child's taking its first breath. (B), (C), and (D) are incorrect.

610. **The answer is B.** (Mosby, *Obstetrical and Neonatal Emergencies.*) (B) Immediately perform intubation and prepare to suction the trachea clear of all meconium. The intubation procedure should be repeated until all meconium has been cleared. No ventilations should be administered between intubations. (A) Although 100 percent oxygen by "blow by" is indicated, it is not definitive care for this patient. (C) Ventilation with a bag-valve-mask would force meconium into the lower airways and cause possible aspiration pneumonia. (D) Stimulation would possibly increase respiratory effort, therefore increasing the risk of aspiration.

611. **The answer is A.** (Brady, *Emergency Management of the Neonate.*) This child has a 1-minute Apgar score of 7. The combination of a pink body and cyanotic extremities scores 1. The pulse rate over 100 scores 2. The grimace scores 1. Some flexion of the extremities scores 1, and a strong cry scores 2. It is suggested that the Paramedic be very familiar with Apgar scoring. Apgar scoring is performed at 1 minute and 5 minutes after birth. (B), (C), and (D) are incorrect.

612. **The answer is A.** (Brady, *Emergency Management of the Neonate.*) (A) A premature infant is one who is born prior to 38 weeks' gestation or weighs less than 2500 g. Premature neonates are prone to respiratory disorders, hypothermia, volume depletion, and cardio-vascular problems. (B), (C), and (D) are incorrect.

613. **The answer is C.** (Mosby/ACEP, *The Critical Pediatric Patient.*) Using the inverted pyramid, the steps in the resuscitation of a newborn are drying, warming, stimulating, and suction-ing followed by (C) the administration of oxygen, then (B) ventilation via bag-valve-mask, then (A) chest compressions, and finally (D) the administration of medications.

614. **The answer is D.** (Caroline, *Neonatal Care and Transport.*) (D) A breech presentation can create special problems during the birth of the neonate, but it is a problem that occurs, not during pregnancy, but during actual childbirth. (A) Antepartum hemorrhage, (B) pre-eclampsia, and (C) multiple pregnancy are all factors that may affect the neonate at birth.

615. **The answer is D.** (Mosby, *Obstetric and Neonatal Emergencies.*) The umbilical cord con-tains three vessels: two arteries and one vein. Cannulation of the umbilical vein is an excel-lent pathway for the delivery of medication to the neonate. (A), (B), and (C) are incorrect.

616. **The answer is B.** (Brady, *Emergency Management of the Neonate.*) The neonate who is hypovolemic for any reason (e.g., dehydration due to vomiting, diarrhea, or hemorrhage) should receive 10 mL/kg of a volume expander to increase intravascular volume. In this example, volume expanders include whole blood, albumin, Ringer's lactate, and normal saline solution. (A) and (C) are incorrect. (D) is the correct volume for a child over 1 month of age.

617. **The answer is D.** (Brady, *Emergency Management of the Neonate.*) The neonatal dose of naloxone (Narcan) is 0.01 mg/kg. Keep in mind that this dosage is only for infants less than 1 month of age. Children over the age of 1 month use a different dosing regimen. (A), (B), and (C) are incorrect values for the neonate.

PEDIATRICS

Directions: Each item below contains four suggested responses. Select the **one best** response to each item.

618. The pediatric age group most likely to suffer from fear of blood and mutilation is
  (A) school-aged children (6–11 years)
  (B) infants and toddlers (birth to 3 years)
  (C) adolescents (12–18 years)
  (D) preschoolers (4–5 years)

619. The pediatric age group most likely to suffer from separation anxiety is
  (A) school-aged children (6–11 years)
  (B) infants and toddlers (birth to 3 years)
  (C) adolescents (12–18 years)
  (D) preschoolers (4–5 years)

620. In pediatric emergencies, the Paramedic must deal with the child's care giver as well as with the patient. Which of the following actions would be beneficial in managing the child's care giver?

  (A) Explain to the care giver that you must do your job and he or she must leave.
  (B) Tell the care giver to relax and you will take care of everything.
  (C) Give the care giver a role in assisting in the care of the child.
  (D) Have a spouse or family member remove the care giver from the room.

621. When the Paramedic is treating an adolescent patient, it is important to

(A) Discuss all interventions with the patient and allow them input into their treatment.

(B) Discuss all interventions with the parent, and inform the patient of the parent's decision.

(C) Inform the adolescent that your interventions are necessary and they must agree to the treatment protocol.

(D) Transport the patient without intervention if they become disagreeable with your treatments due to lack of information.

622. Which of the following are normal vital signs for a 6-month-old child?

(A) pulse 100–160, systolic blood pressure 50–75, respiration 30–60

(B) pulse 90–120, systolic blood pressure 80–100, respiration 25–40

(C) pulse 60–90, systolic blood pressure 90–120, respiration 15–20

(D) pulse 70–110, systolic blood pressure 80–110, respiration 18–25

623. Which of the following are normal vital signs for a 3-year-old child?

(A) pulse 80–120, systolic blood pressure 80–110, respiration 20–30

(B) pulse 90–120, systolic blood pressure 80–100, respiration 25–40

(C) pulse 60–90, systolic blood pressure 90–120, respiration 15–20

(D) pulse 100–160, systolic blood pressure 50–70, respiration 30–60

624. In infants and small children, the physical assessment should be conducted

(A) head to toe, as in the adult

(B) only if absolutely necessary

(C) toe to head

(D) only in the areas affected by illness or injury

625. You are on the scene of a pediatric patient with difficulty breathing. Your partner forgot the pediatric blood pressure cuff in the vehicle and is taking the patient's blood pressure with an adult cuff. What would be an appropriate response to this intervention?

(A) Inform your partner that it is inappropriate to obtain pediatric blood pressure with an adult cuff.

(B) Accept your partner's blood pressure reading as accurate.

(C) Reduce the systolic by 10 mmHg due to cuff size.

(D) Estimate the patient's blood pressure using pulse points.

626. In obtaining the pulse rate of the pediatric patient, the Paramedic should monitor the patient's pulse for at least how many seconds?

(A) 15

(B) 30

(C) 45

(D) 60

627. All of the following are common types of fractures found in the pediatric patient EXCEPT

(A) comminuted fractures

(B) bend fractures

(C) buckle fractures

(D) greenstick fractures

628. Which of the following is NOT a factor in the intubation of the pediatric patient?

(A) The tongue is larger in relation to the remainder of the upper airway.
(B) The cricoid ring has the smallest diameter of all the airway structures.
(C) The tracheal cartilage is hard and bony, allowing for easier intubation.
(D) The smaller structures of the larynx and trachea make visualization more difficult.

629. Bronchiolitis, a viral infection, is most commonly seen in which pediatric age group?

(A) 6–12 months old
(B) 1–3 years old
(C) 3–5 years old
(D) 6–12 years old

630. You respond to a call for a child with difficulty breathing. On your arrival, you find a male child, about 3 years old. He is sitting in a tripod position, in the sniffing position with his chin thrust upward. His mother explains that he was fine this morning and then developed a high fever and cannot speak. The child looks extremely scared, and you notice he will not swallow and is drooling. The most appropriate diagnosis is

(A) croup
(B) foreign-body obstruction
(C) caustic ingestion
(D) epiglottitis

631. You respond to a call for a "child not breathing." On your arrival, the mother is hysterical and tells you that she placed the child in for a nap about an hour ago. When she went to wake him, he was not responsive and she called 911. She states that the child is 4 months old and has been perfectly healthy. You begin CPR and transport the child to the hospital. The most appropriate cause of the child's condition is

(A) sudden infant death syndrome
(B) child abuse
(C) choking
(D) an undiagnosed respiratory infection

632. In the case of a SIDS event where the child has obviously been dead for several hours and is cold and lifeless, the main responsibility of the Paramedic is

(A) Begin CPR and transport the child.
(B) Tell the parents what they should have done to help prior to your arrival.
(C) Assist the parents in their grief and offer to contact relatives, priest or rabbi, or family and friends.
(D) Notify the police department and leave the premises after you have done the appropriate paperwork.

633. All of the following factors have been identified to cause seizures in the pediatric patient EXCEPT

(A) Reye's syndrome
(B) fever
(C) trauma
(D) dysrhythmia

634. The Paramedic's initial action in the treatment of the seizing child is

(A) Administer diazepam 0.3 mg/kg IV.
(B) Administer 25 percent dextrose 1 mL/kg IV.
(C) Establish airway.
(D) Administer 100 percent oxygen.

635. You are called to the scene of a 6-month-old child with a high fever and lethargy. On your arrival, the father explains that the child has had a recent upper respiratory infection and ear infection. Your examination of the child reveals that the child is irritable, with high fever, lethargy, and a bulging anterior fontanelle. The father also states that the child has not been eating well at all. You suspect

(A) epiglottitis
(B) croup
(C) bronchiolitis
(D) meningitis

636. Which of the following children is having the most severe asthma attack?

(A) a 7-year-old with mild end-expiratory wheezes who is awake and alert
(B) a 6-year-old who has loud wheezes in all fields and is lethargic
(C) a 9-year-old who is in the tripod position, is lethargic, has wheezes in all lung fields, and has accessory muscle use
(D) a 6-year-old who is sleepy, has a silent chest, and has accessory muscle use

637. Which of the following is not a beta$_2$-adrenergic agonist used in the treatment of pediatric asthma?

(A) methylprednisolone
(B) epinephrine
(C) albuterol
(D) terbutaline

638. The most common dysrhythmia found in the pediatric patient is

(A) supraventricular tachycardia
(B) ventricular tachycardia
(C) asystole
(D) bradycardia

639. All of the following children should receive a rapid cardiopulmonary assessment to recognize and prevent decompensation and cardiac arrest EXCEPT

(A) a 6-year-old with a heart rate of 58
(B) a 6-year-old with respiratory distress and cyanosis
(C) a 6-year-old with a closed fracture of the radius and/or ulna
(D) a 6-year-old with an open femur fracture

640. Which of the following people would most likely fit the description of a person capable of child abuse?

(A) an unemployed factory worker
(B) a decorated police captain
(C) a caring mother of four children
(D) all of the above

641. All of the following are common injuries that suggest an abused child EXCEPT

(A) a wrist fracture in a 6-year-old in which the mother states "he fell off his bicycle"
(B) injuries in various stages of healing
(C) obvious fractures in children less than 2 years old
(D) bruises or burns with particular patterns

642. You respond to a call for an unconscious child. Upon your arrival, you find an 8-year-old female unconscious with an open head injury in the occipital region. Further investigation reveals greenish-yellow facial bruising in the orbital area as well as various bruises on her arms and legs. Upon questioning, the father states that the child was playing near the top of the stairs and fell down on her head. Your number one priority should be to

(A) Stabilize the child's cervical spine and assess the ABCs.
(B) Further question the father about the abusive injury pattern.
(C) Have your partner care for the child while you hold the father until police arrive.
(D) Contact medical control for instructions.

643. Intraosseous infusion is indicated for pediatric patients who are in need of fluid replacement but in whom no peripheral IV can be established. The intraosseous needle may be safely inserted in patients up to

(A) 3 years of age
(B) 4 years of age
(C) 5 years of age
(D) 6 years of age

644. Volume replacement for the hypotensive pediatric patient should include an initial fluid bolus of

(A) 10 mL/kg
(B) 15 mL/kg
(C) 20 mL/kg
(D) 25 mL/kg

645. The initial pediatric dose of IV or intraosseous epinephrine in asystole is

(A) 1.0 mg of a 1:10,000 solution
(B) 0.1 mg/kg of a 1:10,000 solution
(C) 0.01 mg/kg of a 1:10,000 solution
(D) 0.1 mg/kg of a 1:1,000 solution

646. The initial dose of atropine in pediatric bradycardia is

(A) 2.0 mg/kg
(B) 0.2 mg/kg
(C) 0.02 mg/kg
(D) 0.02 mcg/kg

647. The definition of bradycardia in an infant is

(A) heart rate less than 60 beats per minute
(B) heart rate less than 70 beats per minute
(C) heart rate less than 80 beats per minute
(D) heart rate less than 90 beats per minute

PEDIATRICS

ANSWERS

618. The answer is D. (Mosby/ACEP, *Pediatric Assessment.*) (D) Preschool-aged children have simplistic fears and may take the comments made by emergency medical services providers literally. They have fears of abandonment, darkness, and unknown situations as well as blood and mutilation. With this in mind, the Paramedic should choose words carefully so as to not "imply" something to the child. (A), (B), and (C) are incorrect.

619. The answer is B. (Mosby/ACEP, *Pediatric Assessment.*) (B) Infants and toddlers are prone to separation anxiety as well as fear of strangers. It is wise to let the children sit on their parent's lap while examining them. In addition, examinations should be rapid and limited to pertinent areas of the chief complaint. (A), (C), and (D) are incorrect.

620. The answer is C. (Brady, *General Approach to Pediatric Assessment.*) (C) The Paramedic can decrease the stress of the care giver by allowing him or her to assist in the care of the child. There is often a feeling of guilt involved when a child becomes sick or injured. Allowing the care giver to become active in the care of the child will alleviate this guilt. In addition, it will give the Paramedic a valuable patient care tool to assist in calming the child. (A) will only serve to cause additional tension and upset the child. Although (B) may work in some situations, it does nothing to assist the care giver in dealing with the illness or injury of the child. (D) is inappropriate unless the care giver is unable to control his or her emotions and will hinder the care of the child.

621. The answer is A. (Mosby, *Pediatrics.*) (A) Adolescents have fear of loss of control as well as altered body image. If the Paramedic allows the adolescent to have input in his or her care, this will serve to alleviate his or her fears and assist the Paramedic in properly performing his or her duties. (B) Although the parent should definitely be involved in the decision-making process, the adolescent should also have a good degree of input into the treatment. (C) Informed consent is a legal issue, and the adolescent should be informed that treatments exist to help them; however, in this situation, the Paramedic is offering no choice to the patient. (D) All patients should be treated for illness. Treatments should be completely explained to the patients prior to their initiation. This type of activity will serve to increase the overall quality of patient care.

622. **The answer is B.** (Brady, *General Approach to Pediatric Assessment.*) (B) would be the most appropriate vitals sign set for the 6-month-old. (A) would be the normal range of vital signs for the newborn. (C) is the normal range of vital signs for children over 10 years of age. (D) gives the normal vital signs for a 6-year-old patient.

623. **The answer is A.** (Brady, *General Approach to Pediatric Assessment.*) (A) would be the most appropriate vital signs for the 3-year-old child. (B) would be most appropriate for the 6-month-old child. (C) would be most appropriate for the 10-year-old child, and (D) would be most appropriate for a newborn.

624. **The answer is C.** (Caroline, *Pediatric Emergencies.*) (C) The pediatric assessment for a child between infancy and 24 months old should be conducted from toe to head. Small children generally do not like their faces touched. If the Paramedic begins the assessment at the head, this may cause the child to become apprehensive about the remainder of the examination. (A), (B), and (D) are incorrect.

625. **The answer is A.** (Brady, *General Approach to Pediatric Assessment.*) (A) You must inform your partner that it is inappropriate to obtain pediatric vital signs with adult equipment. This type of assessment is not accurate. Your partner should be instructed to use the proper equipment. (B) is incorrect because your responsibility is to the patient. Accepting inaccurate readings is not in your patient's best interest. (C) is incorrect. There is no formula for using an adult cuff on a pediatric patient. (D) Although some estimation using pulse points is mildly accurate, this is not a proven method in obtaining pediatric vital signs.

626. **The answer is B.** (Brady, *General Approach to Pediatric Assessment.*) (B) Due to variations in pulse rate during respirations, the Paramedic should assess the pulse for no less than 30 seconds at the carotid or radial pulse points. (A), (C), and (D) are incorrect.

627. **The answer is A.** (Brady, *General Approach to Pediatric Assessment.*) (A) Comminuted fractures are not commonly seen in pediatric patients. (B) Bend fractures (angulation and deformity with break), (C) buckle fractures (raised or bulging projection at fracture site), and (D) greenstick fractures (incomplete break in the bone) are all common and due to the softness of the bone because of growth plates being open.

628. **The answer is C.** (Mosby/ACEP, *Pediatric Assessment.*) (C) The tracheal cartilage in a child is softer and may hinder intubation attempts due to its texture. (A), (B), and (D) are all factors that may hinder intubation attempts in the child.

629. The answer is A. (Mosby, *Pediatrics*.) (A) Bronchiolitis is most commonly seen in the 6- to 12-month-old child. This viral infection, commonly caused by the respiratory syncytial virus, is characterized by an upper respiratory infection that presents similarly to an asthmatic attack. (B), (C), and (D) are incorrect.

630. The answer is D. (Caroline, *Pediatric Emergencies*.) (D) Epiglottitis usually presents in children between the ages of 2 and 6 years old. It is a bacterial infection characterized by an abrupt onset of high fever, severe sore throat, difficulty swallowing, drooling, tripod positioning, and muffled speech. This is a true emergency, and the Paramedic should identify this infection and transport immediately. (A) Croup is a viral infection characterized by a low-grade fever and seal-type bark. (B) and (C) are also incorrect.

631. The answer is A. (Caroline, *Pediatric Emergencies*.) (A) Sudden infant death syndrome (SIDS) affects approximately 10,000 infants a year in the United States. This is an unexplained event that occurs in otherwise healthy infants. It is typical that the child is put to sleep and the parent finds the child not breathing and pulseless. The cause of SIDS is generally unknown; however, it may be connected with sleep position. Autopsy reveals no apparent causative agent for the child's death. (B) Child abuse may also cause the Paramedic to find a lifeless child in bed, but there are usually signs suggestive of such abuse. (C) Choking is usually associated with a foreign body and is not usually connected with a sleeping child. (D) Although a respiratory infection may cause respiratory distress and failure, in this case the mother stated the child was otherwise healthy. Historically, this is not the cause of the cardiac arrest.

632. The answer is C. (Caroline, *Pediatric Emergencies*.) (C) In cases where a child is obviously dead and no CPR effort has been begun, the Paramedic should turn his or her attention to the parents. The parents have now become the patients, since they are suffering from overwhelming emotional grief as well as feelings of guilt and helplessness. They need assistance in dealing with this type of loss, and it is the Paramedic's job to provide such assistance. (A) Although in some cases CPR may be appropriate as psychological first aid to the parents, in this case it would be futile and meaningless. (B) will only serve to reinforce the parents' already overwhelming feelings of guilt. (D) constitutes abandonment on the part of the Paramedic, since the parents have now become the patients.

633. The answer is D. (Brady, *Pediatric Medical Emergencies*.) (D) Dysrhythmias are not a causative factor in pediatric seizures.(A) Reye's syndrome, which has no identified etiological factor, will cause seizure in late stages. (B) Fever is a common cause of seizure in pediatric patients. (C) Trauma, specifically, head trauma, is a causative factor in seizures in pediatric patients as well as in adults.

634. The answer is C. (Caroline, *Pediatric Emergencies*.) (C) The establishment of a patent airway is the most important factor in the treatment of the pediatric seizure patient. After the airway is established, the administration of 100 percent oxygen is necessary to maintain oxygenation of the patient during the seizure. The Paramedic should remember that most pediatric deaths from seizures are secondary to hypoxia. Although (A) and (B) are interventions not above the level of the Paramedic, they are not the initial actions.

635. **The answer is D.** (Brady, *Pediatric Emergencies.*) (D) Meningitis in children may be viral (aseptic), which is usually self-limiting, or bacterial. The child with meningitis will present with high fever, headache, joint pain, photophobia, poor feeding, and, in the case of the infant, bulging fontanelle due to meningeal swelling. Treatment is supportive, with fluid replacement indicated for dehydration. (A), (B), and (C) are incorrect.

636. **The answer is D.** (Caroline, *Pediatric Emergencies.*) (D) The child with the silent chest, an ominous sign in any asthmatic, is certainly the most serious case. Any asthmatic with a silent chest needs rapid intervention to produce adequate ventilation and tidal volume. A silent chest is indicative of extremely narrowed airways and is life threatening. The patient in case (A) is not critical, but interventions must be attempted to prevent this patient from decompensating. (B) and (C) represent serious cases that require immediate intervention.

637. **The answer is A.** (Mosby, *Pediatrics.*) (A) Methylprednisolone, although used in the treatment of asthmatic patients, is not a beta$_2$-adrenergic agonist. Methylprednisolone (Solu-Medrol) is classified as a corticosteroid. (B), (C), and (D) are all beta$_2$-adrenergic agonists.

638. **The answer is D.** (Brady, *Pediatric Emergencies.*) (D) Bradycardia is by far the most common dysrhythmia found in the pediatric patient. It results from hypoxia, hypotension, and acidosis. (A) Supraventricular tachycardia, although not common, may be seen in the pediatric patient. (B) Ventricular tachycardia is rarely seen in pediatric patients unless that patient has a congenital abnormality. (C) Asystole is a common cardiac arrest rhythm encountered in pediatric patients. Most commonly, the child in respiratory distress will develop bradycardia and then degenerate into asystole.

639. **The answer is C.** (Brady, *Pediatric Emergencies.*) (C) A 6-year-old with a closed fracture of the radius and/or ulna does not meet the criteria for rapid cardiopulmonary assessment unless the mechanism of injury suggests hidden injury. This is an isolated injury that usually does not result in critical decompensation. (A), (B), and (D) are all instances in which a rapid cardiopulmonary assessment should be done to prevent cardiopulmonary arrest.

640. **The answer is D.** (Brady, *Pediatric Emergencies.*) (D) Child abusers come from all geographic, economic, religious, occupational, and educational backgrounds. The typical child abuser could possibly be under financial, marital, or occupational stress. In addition, the child abuser may have been abused as a child.

641. **The answer is A.** (Mosby, *Pediatrics.*) (A) The child with an isolated wrist fracture does not immediately fall into the category of child abuse. Wrist fractures are commonly seen in injuries sustained from falls, and the statement of the mother indicates a very possible

scenario. (B), (C), and (D) are all indicative of abuse patterns and should be investigated further. The Paramedic should keep in mind that the main priority is the treatment of the child and not the questioning or accusation of the parents or care givers.

642. The answer is A. (Mosby, *Pediatrics.*) (A) Stabilization of the child's cervical spine and the ABCs constitute the Paramedic's first priority. Once you have determined the severity and cause of the injury, it is not necessary to (B) question the parent suspiciously. Treat the patient, and report suspicions of illegal activity to law enforcement personnel. The Paramedic should not attempt to (C) hold the suspect until the police arrive. (D) Although consulting medical control is always an option, maintenance of the airway and stabilization of the cervical spine are the highest priorities.

643. The answer is D. (Mosby, *Pediatrics.*) (D) Intraosseous infusion should be used in patients 6 years of age or younger. It is indicated when attempts at peripheral access have failed and the patient is unconscious. Some indications are severe shock, cardiac arrest, status asthmaticus, and prolonged seizures. (A), (B), and (C) are incorrect.

644. The answer is C. (Brady, *Pediatric Emergencies.*) The initial volume replacement for the pediatric patient is 20 mL/kg. This infusion is used for dehydration, hypovolemia, and any other disease or trauma process that would cause hypotension secondary to fluid loss in the pediatric patient.

645. The answer is C. (Brady, *Pediatric Emergencies.*) (C) In cases of asystole, the initial pediatric dosage of epinephrine is 0.01 mg/kg of a 1:10,000 solution. (A), (B), and (D) are incorrect, although answer (D) is the initial endotracheal dose of epinephrine in asystole.

646. The answer is C. (Brady, *Pediatric Emergencies.*) The initial dose of atropine in cases of bradycardia in the pediatric patient is 0.02 mg/kg. The minimum individual dose is 0.1 mg, and the maximum individual dose is 0.5 mg for a child and 1.0 mg for an adolescent. (A), (B), and (D) are incorrect.

647. The answer is C. (Brady, *Pediatric Emergencies.*) (C) Bradycardia in an infant is defined as a heart rate less than 80 beats per minute. The definition of bradycardia in a child is less than 60 beats per minute. (A), (B), and (D) are incorrect.

GERIATRICS

Directions: Each item below contains four suggested responses. Select the **one best** response to each item.

648. All of the following statements are true about the difficulties in assessing the geriatric patient EXCEPT

(A) The geriatric patient may fail to report initial symptoms.

(B) The geriatric patient has a lack of temperature-regulatory mechanisms.

(C) Emotional factors may make geriatric assessment difficult.

(D) Many geriatric patients suffer from several chronic problems, making diagnosis more difficult.

649. You respond to an 83-year-old male who has been disoriented for a few days. Upon your arrival, you find that the patient has been complaining of seeing a yellow haze and is just "not feeling right." At the hospital, the patient is diagnosed with digitalis toxicity. All of the following are common accidental causes of medication reactions in the elderly patient EXCEPT

(A) Geriatric patients have changes in drug absorption and metabolism.

(B) Geriatric patients may see more than one physician and have duplicate medications.

(C) Due to memory deterioration, the geriatric patient may accidentally overdose on medication.

(D) Geriatric patients use medications in an attempt to end their lives.

650. Which of the following is the number one cause of decreased cardiac output in the otherwise healthy geriatric patient?

(A) deterioration of the electrical conduction system of the heart
(B) arteriosclerosis
(C) hypertension
(D) cardiac hypertrophy

651. Which of the following is NOT a typical age-related physiological change?

(A) increase in brain mass
(B) decreased respiratory vital capacity
(C) decreased renal function
(D) degeneration of the joints

652. All of the following are common complaints in the elderly EXCEPT

(A) fatigue
(B) dizziness
(C) chest pain
(D) falls

653. You are dispatched to an 81-year-old female who has fallen on the sidewalk. On your arrival, you find the woman lying on the ground, alert, and oriented. You notice a large hematoma in the occipital region with little external bleeding. Which of the following would lead you to a high index of suspicion for brain injury in this patient?

(A) Based on mental status, there is no evidence of brain injury.
(B) Due to decreased brain mass, elderly patients are prone to head injuries.
(C) Little external bleeding with a hematoma usually means it is bleeding internally.
(D) The occipital region is prone to internal injuries.

654. You respond to a 75-year-old male with a syncopal episode. On your arrival, you find the male awake and lying on a couch. The patient has a heart rate of 40 beats per minute, a blood pressure of 90/76, and a respiratory rate of 20 breaths per minute. The patient states that he is okay when lying down but feels faint when he stands. In fact, he passed out before. You acquire an ECG, which shows a third-degree heart block. The type of syncope associated with heart blocks is known as

(A) cardiogenic syncope
(B) Stokes-Adams syncope
(C) psychogenic syncope
(D) orthostatic syncope

655. Your patient is a 72-year-old female who has just suffered a seizure. Upon arrival, you find that the patient is postictal. Family members on the scene tell you that she has no history of medical problems and is quite physically fit. As a matter of fact, she fell and hit her head recently while rollerblading and got right back up and continued skating. Based on this information, what would be the most likely cause of this seizure activity?

(A) alcohol withdrawal
(B) hypoglycemia
(C) epilepsy
(D) subdural hematoma

656. You arrive at a well-kept residence to find an 82-year-old woman who has multiple bruises about her face and arms. The family members who are present state that she has been a burden and has been falling constantly. The patient, who is alert and answers your questions, states that they are trying to kill her and hit her all the time. The family states that she is senile and has no idea what she is talking about. After medically treating the patient, the Paramedic may suspect

(A) The patient suffers from senile dementia.
(B) The patient is a victim of elder abuse.
(C) The patient is embarrassed about her falls and is confabulating a story.
(D) The patient may be suffering from head injuries due to the fall.

GERIATRICS

A N S W E R S

648. **The answer is B.** (Mosby/ACEP, *Geriatric Assessment*.) (B) Although the temperature-regulatory mechanism in the geriatric patient may be depressed, geriatric patients do not lack this ability. (A) Geriatric patients are prone to not complain of initial symptoms for fear of hospitalization and other issues. Answer (C) psychological and emotional factors may impede the paramedic from obtaining a good history. Answer (D), because geriatric patients may suffer from several chronic problems, it makes it more difficult for the paramedic to accurately diagnose the etiology of the current problem.

649. **The answer is D.** (Mosby/ACEP, *Geriatric Assessment*.) (D) Although the incidence of suicide in geriatric patients amounts to approximately 25 percent of all suicides, this is not an accidental cause of medication reactions. (A), (B), and (C) are all common causes of accidental medication reactions in the elderly patient.

650. **The answer is D.** (Caroline, *Emergencies in the Elderly*.) (D) Cardiac hypertrophy is enlargement of the cardiac muscle. This is common and naturally occurring in the geriatric patient. Hypertrophy is considered to be caused by stiffening blood vessels. Hypertrophy causes decreased cardiac output even in normally healthy patients. (A), (B), and (C), while all normal in the physiological process of aging, are not the primary causes of decreased cardiac output.

651. **The answer is A.** (Brady, *Emergencies in the Elderly Patient*.) (A) Increase in brain mass is not a normal age-related physiological change. Some age-related changes are decreased brain mass, decreased cardiac stroke volume and rate, (B) decreased respiratory vital capacity, (C) decreased renal function, decreased total body water, and (D) degeneration of the joints.

652. The answer is C. (Brady, *Emergencies in the Elderly.*) Elderly patients generally have common complaints for which they call for assistance. For example, (A) fatigue and (B) dizziness are some of the most common complaints in the elderly patient. (D) Falls are another common complaint, and the Paramedic must be cautious not to rule out other causes that may have lead to the patient's falling (e.g., syncopal events). (C) Due to decreased nerve conduction velocity and deterioration of the nervous system, many elderly patients may have no complaint of chest pain, even during a cardiac event. Paramedics should be alert to other signs and symptoms of cardiac events in these cases.

653. The answer is B. (Brady, *Emergencies in the Elderly.*) (B) is correct. Elderly patients are prone to severe internal head injuries due to decreased brain mass. This allows free movement of the brain in the cranial cavity, increasing the incidence of injury. In addition, the patient cannot be diagnosed on (A) mental status alone because brain injuries in the elderly, especially bleeding, may not be symptomatic due to increased capacity of the cranial cavity, which may lead to the delay of signs of increasing intercranial pressure. (C) and (D) are incorrect.

654. The answer is B. (Brady, *Emergencies in the Elderly Patient.*) (B) Stokes-Adams syncope is commonly associated with heart blocks, and the patient will generally not produce enough cardiac output to support a stable mental status. This patient, when lying down, will have enough perfusion to remain conscious, but the decreased cardiac output due to the heart block will not produce enough perfusion to the brain while standing. (D) Orthostatic syncope usually occurs due to decreased hypovolemic states, which are commonly caused by dehydration, certain medications, and prolonged bed rest. (A) and (C) are incorrect.

655. The answer is D. (Mosby/ACEP, *Geriatric Assessment.*) (D) Based on the patient's history in this scenario, this patient is most likely suffering from a subdural hematoma. Due to increased capacity of the cranial cavity, geriatric patients may be slow to develop symptoms from bleeding in the head. (A) Although alcohol withdrawal, (B) hypoglycemia, and (C) epilepsy are all common causes of seizure in the elderly, there is no significant historical information that can support these diagnoses. Other causes of new-onset seizures can be mass lesions and stroke.

656. The answer is B. (Mosby/ACEP, *Geriatric Assessment.*) (B) Elder abuse knows no socioeconomic boundaries. This patient has appeared to you in a properly alert fashion and answered your questions correctly. Her story of abuse should not be disregarded due to statements from family members. Paramedics must remember that the geriatric patient is the patient and should be questioned about her or his condition. Although (A) senile dementia and (C) confabulation are real scenarios, this patient is awake and alert. (D) Subdural bleeding in this case may be possible, but mental status and injury patterns suggest otherwise.

ABUSE AND ASSAULT

Directions: Each item below contains four suggested responses. Select the **one best** response to each item.

657. All of the following are categories of abuse EXCEPT

(A) child abuse
(B) sexual abuse
(C) elderly abuse
(D) drug abuse

658. All of the following are characteristics associated with the profile of a typical adult abuser EXCEPT

(A) poorly educated
(B) frequently jealous, irritable, and explosive
(C) usually outgoing and very sociable
(D) likely alcohol and drug user

659. You are waved down by a young child who requests that you please come and help his mother, who is bleeding. Upon your entering the patient's apartment, you find a 40-year-old female holding her right arm, with multiple facial bruises and active bleeding from the mouth. The patient's husband has alcohol on his breath and claims that his wife slipped on the floor and hit herself on the kitchen table. As you begin to assess the patient and treat her wounds, you are very suspicious that this may represent an example of

(A) child abuse
(B) adult abuse
(C) geriatric abuse
(D) drug abuse

660. Which of the following is the correct percentage of women who visit emergency departments for the treatment of symptoms related to abuse annually?

(A) 5 percent
(B) 10 percent
(C) 35 percent
(D) 75 percent

661. You are sent to the home of a 77-year-old male who has been injured. As you walk into the house, a younger man who claims to be the patient's son greets you. He has alcohol on his breath and proceeds to tell you that the patient has fallen and hit his chin on the desk. He also tells you that his father is losing his memory, is often combative, and is incontinent of urine day and night. He tells you that he has lost his job recently and is unable to look for another one because of his father's condition. He then begins to become angry and rants about being sick and tired of babysitting his father. When you finally are led to the patient, you find him lying in bed, disheveled, confused, with a swollen and ecchymotic left chin, as well as red finger marks on his right cheek. As you approach the patient, he withdraws from you and proceeds to cover his head with his arms. He also is grossly incontinent of urine. Which of the following best describes this presentation?

(A) child abuse
(B) drug abuse
(C) elder abuse
(D) adult abuse

662. All of the following are characteristics of a typical abuser of the elder EXCEPT

(A) usually does not allow the elder to visit alone with a health care provider
(B) frequently abuses alcohol and drugs
(C) happy, content, and not under any stress
(D) usually does not have any financial responsibility for the elder

663. You are dispatched to an injured 3-year-old boy. As you arrive at the child's home, his 7-year-old sister leads you to the child. She states that her mother is busy washing clothes and her father is at work. As you enter the room, you notice that the child is sitting on the floor, with several bruises on his arms and legs. All of the following are consistent with this representing a case of child abuse EXCEPT

(A) The child only has fresh bruises, without any old scars or burns.
(B) The child seems apathetic and does not cry, even with examination of the bruises.
(C) The child's mother approaches you and demonstrates little interest in her child.
(D) The child's sister states that he has always been a little slow and that he gets hurt a lot.

664. All of the following are typical characteristics of an abusive parent EXCEPT

(A) usually offers a clear, detailed description of each injury to the child

(B) often does not demonstrate any cuddling or closeness to the child

(C) acts abusively often in response to stresses or losses, such as loss of a job or a divorce

(D) frequently involved with alcohol or drugs

665. You are dispatched to a 26-year-old female who has been sexually assaulted. As you arrive at the patient's apartment, you find the patient crying and very upset. She states that a man must have followed her home and quickly put his foot in her apartment door just after she opened it. Then, using the threat of a knife, he raped her. All of the following are parts of the approach to treating this patient EXCEPT

(A) Examine the patient for any signs of serious trauma.

(B) Only examine the patient's vaginal area if she is heavily bleeding.

(C) Attempt to gather any evidence of the patient's sexual assault, such as blood-stained clothing.

(D) Always allow and encourage the patient to shower and use the bathroom to clean up before going to the hospital.

666. All of the following are parts of the correct method of documenting the ambulance call report in a suspected rape case EXCEPT

(A) State, in the patient's own words, exactly what occurred.

(B) Carefully describe the patient's appearance and emotional state.

(C) Carefully document the patient's injuries.

(D) Complete the report by offering your opinion as to whether the patient has or has not been raped.

ABUSE AND ASSAULT

657. The answer is D. (Mosby/ACEP, *Issues of Personal Violence*; Caroline/Little Brown, *Behavioral and Psychiatric Emergencies*.) (A), (B), (C), and adult abuse are some of the categories of abuse. Domestic violence is another frequently used term to describe the use of force by one family member against another with the intent to inflict harm or even death. (D) is incorrect because, even though it may be abusive behavior toward oneself, it is not considered a category of abuse. Abuse is primarily considered as being perpetrated by one individual upon another.

658. The answer is C. (Mosby/ACEP, *Issues of Personal Violence*.) (A), (B), and (D) are correct. (B) is incorrect because an adult abuser usually lacks self-confidence and is socially isolated.

659. The answer is B. (Mosby/ACEP, *Issues of Personal Violence*.) (B) is correct. It may also be referred to as spousal abuse. (A), (C), and (D) are incorrect.

660. The answer is C. (Mosby/ACEP, *Issues of Personal Violence*.) (C) is correct, even though as few as 5 percent of these women are identified.

661. The answer is C. (Mosby/ACEP, *Geriatric Assessment*.) (C) is correct. The four main types of elder abuse are physical abuse, physical neglect, psychological abuse, and material abuse. This presentation demonstrates the first three. (A), (B), and (D) are all incorrect.

662. The answer is D. (Mosby/ACEP, *Issues of Personal Violence*.) (A), (B), and (C) are correct. (D) is incorrect because frequently the elder is financially dependent on the abuser.

663. **The answer is A.** (Caroline/Little Brown, *Pediatric Emergencies.*) (B), (C), and (D) are correct. (A) is incorrect because usually an abused child demonstrates evidence of old scars, burns, or deformities in addition to the new injuries.

664. **The answer is A.** (Caroline/Little Brown, *Pediatric Emergencies.*) (B), (C), and (D) are correct. (A) is incorrect because the abusive parent usually is evasive and offers very little information about what happened to the child.

665. **The answer is D.** (Caroline/Little Brown, *Gynecologic Emergencies.*) (A), (B), and (C) are correct. (D) is incorrect because, if at all possible, you should gently encourage the patient not to use the bathroom or shower, so that emergency department personnel are better able to gather evidence for the police.

666. **The answer is D.** (Caroline/Little Brown, *Gynecologic Emergencies.*) (A), (B), and (C) are correct. (D) is incorrect because, since the ambulance call report is a legal document, you should never offer your opinion as to whether the patient was or was not raped.

ACUTE INTERVENTIONS FOR CHRONIC CARE PATIENTS

Directions: Each item below contains four suggested responses. Select the **one best** response to each item.

667. All of the following are categories of vascular access devices utilized in home health care EXCEPT

    (A) arterial lines

    (B) central venous catheters

    (C) implanted ports

    (D) peripheral inserted central catheters

668. All of the following are characteristics of a central venous catheter EXCEPT

    (A) manufactured by Broviac, Hickman, Groshong, or Corcath

    (B) only come with a single lumen

    (C) are tunneled under the subcutaneous tissue to the venous entrance site

    (D) a small cap covering each lumen

669. You are dispatched to a 56-year-old female who is complaining of substernal chest pain. As you approach the patient, she tells you that she has had 2 hours of substernal chest pain radiating down her left arm. She has a history of angina and has not had chest pain as severe as she has experienced today. She also tells you that she had a mastectomy 4 months ago, is in the process of receiving outpatient chemotherapy, and has a Broviac central venous catheter in place. According to your protocol, you have begun ECG monitoring and high-concentration oxygen by nonrebreather face mask, and have administered sublingual nitroglycerin, without relief. You attempt to begin an IV line, but the patient tells you that she has awful veins. Despite additional nitroglycerin, the patient continues to have chest pain and is also short of breath. You have received medical control permission to administer IV 3 mg morphine sulfate. All of the following are parts of the approach to accessing the central venous catheter EXCEPT

(A) Use aseptic technique, with sterile gloves.

(B) Clamp the catheter with a smooth hemostat.

(C) If an infusion is going in one of the multiple lumens, a free lumen may be used.

(D) Never accept advice from a patient, family member, or care giver concerning the use of the catheter.

670. All of the following are possible complications of accessing vascular access devices EXCEPT

(A) dysuria and increased urinary frequency

(B) infection at the catheter's access site

(C) thrombosis in the catheter

(D) air embolism

671. All of the following are possible complications and emergencies associated with patients who have tracheostomies EXCEPT

(A) respiratory distress

(B) skin rash on both arms

(C) sepsis

(D) tracheal stenosis

672. You are dispatched to the home of a 78-year-old male who is having difficulty breathing. However, as you enter the patient's bedroom, you become aware that the patient has a tracheostomy and is connected to a ventilator. The patient's nurse states that the patient has been having an increase in secretions for the past few days. Then, this morning, the patient began to have difficulty breathing. The nurse also stated that she was having difficulty suctioning the patient today. Your assessment reveals that the patient's respiratory rate is 28 breaths per minute, his pulse rate is 120 beats per minute, and his blood pressure is 162/78. In addition, the patient has circumoral and peripheral cyanosis. Which of the following is the best way to proceed in providing emergency care for this patient?

(A) Contact medical control to discuss various treatment options.
(B) Place the patient and the portable ventilator on the stretcher and transport both to the hospital.
(C) Administer 100 percent oxygen by nonrebreather face mask.
(D) Disconnect the patient from the ventilator and begin to ventilate the patient with a bag-valve-mask attached to the tracheostomy tube.

673. All of the following are possible complications occurring with the use of gastrostomy feeding tubes EXCEPT

(A) pulmonary aspiration
(B) dehydration
(C) diarrhea
(D) headache

674. You are sent to the home of an 82-year-old female with bleeding from a gastrostomy tube site. The patient's home health aide tells you that she was in the process of turning the patient when the patient's gastrostomy tube became caught on the bed. The patient then was noted to begin bleeding from the gastrostomy tube sight. Which of the following is the correct way to care for this patient?

(A) Package the patient, and transport her to the hospital.
(B) Try to maneuver the catheter by pushing it further into the abdomen.
(C) Try to flush the gastrostomy tube with 500 mL saline solution.
(D) Apply direct pressure with a sterile dressing to the bleeding site.

ACUTE INTERVENTIONS FOR CHRONIC CARE PATIENTS

A N S W E R S

667. The answer is A. (Mosby/ACEP, *Specialized Adjuncts for Therapy.*) (B), (C), and (D) are correct. (A) is incorrect because, while arterial lines are vascular access devices, they are not used in the home health care setting. They are usually accessed only in the hospital setting.

668. The answer is B. (Mosby/ACEP, *Specialized Adjuncts for Therapy.*) (A), (C), and (D) are correct. (B) is incorrect because central venous catheters come in single or multiple lumens.

669. The answer is D. (Mosby/ACEP, *Specialized Adjuncts for Therapy.*) (A), (B), and (C) are correct. (D) is incorrect because you should always be open to accepting advice from the patient, family members, and care givers who have been routinely accessing the catheter.

670. The answer is A. (Mosby/ACEP, *Specialized Adjuncts for Therapy.*) (B), (C), (D), sepsis, and a torn or leaking catheter are all possible complications of accessing vascular access devices.

671. The answer is B. (Mosby/ACEP, *Specialized Adjuncts for Therapy.*) (A), (C), (D), site infection, necrosis, fistula, and subcutaneous or mediastinal emphysema are sometimes complications and emergencies. (B) is incorrect because it has nothing to do with a patient who has a tracheostomy.

672. The answer is D. (Mosby/ACEP, *Specialized Adjuncts for Therapy.*) (D) is correct. (A) is incorrect because, if permitted by your medical control, you should begin to administer advanced life support to the patient with difficulty breathing. (B) is incorrect because the patient is already cyanotic and having difficulty breathing while being connected to the ventilator. (C) is incorrect because administering 100 percent oxygen by nonrebreather face mask is useless, since the patient is breathing through the tracheostomy tube opening in his neck.

673. **The answer is D.** (Mosby/ACEP, *Specialized Adjuncts for Therapy.*) (A), (B), (C), nausea, bacterial contamination, electrolyte imbalance, and tube displacement are all possible complications of gastrostomy tubes. (D) is incorrect.

674. **The answer is D.** (Mosby/ACEP, *Specialized Adjuncts for Therapy.*) (D) is correct. (A) is incorrect because the bleeding site should be treated immediately. (B) is incorrect because a gastrostomy tube should never be pushed further into the abdomen blindly. (C) is incorrect because the bleeding is coming from the gastrostomy tube site, not from inside the stomach. Therefore, flushing the gastrostomy tube is of no benefit.

SECTION VII: OPERATIONS

The following topics are covered in Section VII:

- Ambulance Operations
- Incident Command
- Rescue Awareness
- Hazardous Materials

AMBULANCE OPERATIONS

Directions: Each item below contains four suggested responses. Select the **one best** response to each item.

675. Which of the following is NOT a circumstance in which air medical transport should be considered?

  (A) lengthy extrication times
  (B) lengthy ground transport time
  (C) spinal injury
  (D) lengthy manual transport out of a remote area

676. All of the following patients meet air medical transport criteria EXCEPT

  (A) a 47-year-old male who has suffered a fall of 40 feet while rock climbing
  (B) a 39-year-old female who was thrown from her car in a motor vehicle accident on a desolate highway
  (C) a patient with major trauma who is 30 minutes from the hospital by ground transport
  (D) a 14-year-old male who has overdosed on his mother's hypertension medication

677. Which of the following laws defines the minimum qualifications of those who may perform various health services, defines the skills that each type of practitioner is legally permitted to use, and establishes a means of certification for various categories of health care professionals?

   (A) Medical Practice Act
   (B) Good Samaritan Act
   (C) Negligence Act
   (D) EMS Certification Act

678. You respond to a motor vehicle accident. On your arrival, you find an adult male about 20 years old. The male appears quite intoxicated and is slightly argumentative. He is involved in a one-car collision with a telephone pole. Your partner decides that the patient has no significant injuries, although the patient is complaining of neck pain. You transport the patient to the hospital at his request. However, you do not immobilize the patient, and you transport him seated in the crew chair of your vehicle. The patient is later diagnosed with a cervical spine fracture and is now suffering from paralysis. You and your partner may face charges of

   (A) assault
   (B) battery
   (C) negligence
   (D) slander

679. Based on the 1974 KKK-A-1822 standards, match the following ambulances with the correct description.

   (A) type 1
   (B) type 2
   (C) type 3

   1. Conventional cab and chassis with a modular ambulance body. There is no passageway between the driver's compartment and the patient's compartment.
   2. Specialty van with forward cab and integral body. There is a passageway between the driver's compartment and the patient's compartment.
   3. Van-type vehicle, possibly with a raised roof. There is a passageway between the driver's compartment and the patient's compartment.

AMBULANCE
OPERATIONS

ANSWERS

675. **The answer is C.** (Mosby/ACEP, *Special Situations*.) (C) Spinal injury is not a criterion in itself for air medical transport. However, the patient who may have multiple trauma in addition to spinal injury may fall into the category for air medical transport. (A), (B), and (D) are all criteria for patient removal by air.

676. **The answer is D.** (Mosby/ACEP, *Special Situations*.) (D) A 14-year-old male who has overdosed does not meet air medical transport criteria. This patient should be monitored and taken by ground transport to the closest hospital. (A), (B), and (C) are all critical traumas that easily meet air medical transport criteria.

677. **The answer is A.** (Caroline, *The Prehospital World*.) (A) The Medical Practice Act defines the levels of training and certification as well as the minimum qualifications to become certified at any level of care provider. This act is partially responsible for EMS training curricula at all provider levels. (B) The Good Samaritan Act is a protective act for prehospital providers who render aid in good faith to patients in emergent situations. (C) and (D) are incorrect.

678. **The answer is C.** (Caroline, *The Prehospital World*.) (C) best describes your situation. Negligence occurs when the following conditions are met: (1) there was an injury, (2) the Paramedic had a duty to act, (3) the Paramedic breached that duty to act, and (4) an injury occurred due to that breach of duty. Although the patient was injured prior to the arrival of the crew, aggravation of his injury may have been prevented by early intervention and proper immobilization of the patient. This crew may face charges of negligence for failure to treat the patient in a proper fashion.

679. Answers. (Brady, *The Systems Approach.*)

(A) 1. Type 1 has a conventional cab and chassis with a modular ambulance body. There is no passageway between the driver's compartment and the patient's compartment.

(B) 3. Type 2 is a van-type vehicle, possibly with a raised roof. There is a passageway between the driver's compartment and the patient's compartment.

(C) 2. Type 3 is a specialty van with forward cab and integral body. There is a passageway between the driver's compartment and the patient's compartment.

INCIDENT COMMAND

Directions: Each item below contains four suggested responses. Select the **one best** response to each item.

680. Which of the following is not an objective of the management of a large incident using the incident command system?

(A) It allows all responding agencies to work independently of each other.

(B) It provides an organized plan designed to effectively manage needs.

(C) It defines lines of responsibility and authority.

(D) It offers performance evaluation criteria.

681. Which type of mass casualty incident would be most liable to necessitate the implementation of an emergency operations center as well as secondary levels of management?

(A) a low-impact incident

(B) a high-impact incident

(C) a disaster or catastrophic incident

(D) a terrorist event

682. Define a mass casualty incident.

(A) an incident that can be managed by the initial responding unit

(B) an incident involving large numbers of patients

(C) an incident involving multiple-response agencies

(D) a terrorist event

683. Which of the following is a responsibility of the treatment sector at a major incident?

(A) tagging patients according to their injuries

(B) providing immediate and delayed areas

(C) coordinating procurement of medical supplies from hospitals

(D) establishing a helicopter landing zone

684. The command structure at a major incident can best be described as

(A) a structure in which all sectors have separate commanders who report directly to the communications center

(B) a structure in which a single person is in command of the entire incident with sector commanders reporting their status to the incident commander

(C) a structure with independent commanders representing each agency on the scene

(D) a structure in which commanders are assigned based on patient count

685. You are responding to the scene of a major incident. As a Paramedic, which area should you respond to initially?

(A) triage
(B) treatment
(C) staging
(D) support

686. Upon the identification of a major incident, when should responders identify a command post and incident commander?

(A) immediately upon identification of the incident

(B) upon the arrival of the police department

(C) upon the arrival of the fire department

(D) upon the arrival of a chief officer

687. On the scene of a major incident, you attempt to open a patient's airway and find that he is not breathing. You take the appropriate corrective actions, and there is still no respiratory effort. Using the METTAG system, you should tag this patient

(A) red
(B) yellow
(C) green
(D) black

688. Which of the following is not a component of the START method of triage?

(A) respiratory status
(B) motor status
(C) hemodynamic status
(D) mental status

689. You have begun your assessment of a patient and have found his respiratory system intact, with a respiratory effort under 30 breaths per minute. Using the START method, what should be your next step in the triage of this patient?

(A) transport to the treatment area
(B) assess hemodynamic status
(C) assess mental status
(D) administer oxygen

690. You have completed your hemodynamic status evaluation of a patient, and you are ready to move on to the next step in the START triage method. What would you assess next?

(A) mental status
(B) airway
(C) breathing
(D) motor function

INCIDENT COMMAND

A N S W E R S

680. **The answer is A.** (Brady, *Major Incident Response*.) (A) is incorrect, since it states exactly the opposite of what the incident command system is designed to accomplish. It provides (B) an organized plan to effectively manage needs, (C) a definition of responsibility and authority, and (D) performance evaluation criteria. In addition, it provides a framework that groups similar functions, provides an orderly means of communication, and establishes a common terminology to reduce the probability of confusion during a large incident.

681. **The answer is C.** (Brady, *Major Incident Response*.) (C) A disaster or catastrophic incident will tax the resources of a region and not just the local EMS system. This type of incident will necessitate the implementation of an emergency operations center as well as secondary levels of management. (A) A low-impact incident will usually be handled and mitigated by local EMS responder and does not require mutual aid or assistance from outside agencies. (B) A high-impact incident will necessitate mutual assistance from EMS agencies within the region. (D) Although the probabilities are high that a terrorist incident will probably tax the region in which it occurs, it will not always generate a large patient count; therefore (D) is incorrect.

682. **The answer is B.** (Brady, *Major Incident Response*.) (B) An incident involving large numbers of patients is a mass casualty incident. These incidents are defined in three categories: low impact, high impact, and disaster or catastrophic incident. (A) does not describe a mass casualty incident, since any incident that can be managed by a single unit does not produce large numbers of patients. (C) Mass casualty incidents will most likely involve multiple agencies; however, not all multiple agency responses produce large numbers of patients. (D) Terrorist events may produce large numbers of patients, but some terrorist events are targeted at structures and not people.

683. The answer is B. (Mosby, *Major Incident Response*.) (B) Providing immediate and delayed treatment areas is a direct responsibility of the treatment sector. This allows for the most serious injuries to be treated first. (A) Tagging patients is the responsibility of the triage sector. (C) Procurement of hospital supplies is a responsibility of the support sector. (D) Establishment of the helicopter landing zone is a role of the transportation sector.

684. The answer is B. (Mosby, *Major Incident Response*.) (B) The command structure is based on a single individual who is in control of all operations. This individual will have dedicated commanders in each sector who will generate progress reports to the command post for incident evaluation. (A) is incorrect because sector commanders do not communicate with the communications center. (C) Although each responding agency would probably have a commander with it, those commanders would report to the incident commander for assignment. (D) is incorrect; there is no assignment of commanders based on patient count.

685. The answer is C. (Mosby, *Major Incident Response*.) (C) All responding vehicles and personnel should always report initially to the staging sector for direction. From there they will be assigned to a sector where their resources are needed. (A), (B), and (D) are incorrect.

686. The answer is A. (Brady, *Major Incident Response*.) (A) The first arriving unit, upon identification of a major incident, should set up a command post and direct responding units as well as identify the needs for resources. Command may be passed upon the arrival of a ranking officer; however, the officer may decide to maintain an advisory role to maintain continuity of the initial command structure. (B), (C), and (D) are all incorrect, since the incident command system should be implemented immediately following the identification of a mass casualty incident.

687. The answer is D. (Brady, *Major Incident Response*.) (D) Patients who have no respiratory effort after corrective actions are tagged black (dead or unsalvageable). These incidents do not allow for long-term resuscitative efforts that may use additional resources, making them unavailable to assist other patients. (A), (B), and (C) are incorrect.

688. The answer is B. (Brady, *Major Incident Response*.) (B) The START method of triage evaluates (A) respiratory, (C) hemodynamic, and (D) mental status and does not include the patient's motor status. The patient is evaluated for respiration; if there are no respirations, the patient is marked dead or unsalvageable. If the respirations are above 30 and/or the patient needs airway maintenance, the patient is marked critical/immediate. If the patient has a respiratory rate less than 30, the Paramedic should begin the hemodynamic assessment.

689. The answer is B. (Mosby, *Major Incident Response*.) (B) If your patient's respiratory status is intact and supporting ventilation, you should move on to the hemodynamic assessment. This assessment will consist of monitoring a radial pulse. If the radial pulse is present, then the Paramedic will move on to the assessment of mental status. If a radial pulse is absent, the Paramedic will attempt to control all bleeding and mark the patient immediate. (A) is incorrect, since the patient is not sent to the treatment area until after initial triage is completed. (C) Assessment of mental status is not begun until the completion of hemodynamic assessment. (D) is incorrect. In the triage area, no adjunctive treatment is completed.

690. **The answer is A.** (Brady, *Major Incident Response.*) (A) Mental status is the third step in the START method of triage. If the patient has an impaired mental status and fails to follow simple commands, he or she is marked immediate. If the patient is responsive and alert, he or she is marked delayed. (B) Airway and (C) breathing are both evaluated during the respiratory step of the START method. (D) Motor function is not part of the START method, since mental status is assessed only. The AVPU scale is used in the START method of triage as a mental status indicator.

RESCUE
AWARENESS

Directions: Each item below contains four suggested responses. Select the **one best** response to each item.

691. Identify which of the following is not a part of the Paramedic's primary role at the scene of a rescue operation.

(A) evaluation of scene hazards
(B) securing hazardous materials leaks
(C) gaining access to the patient
(D) extrication of the patient and continued treatment

692. You are operating at a serious collision on a major interstate highway. Traffic flow, although slowed due to the scene, is moving dangerously close to your area of operations. The police officers question you on your feelings toward the safety of the situation. What would be your safest choice in the control of the traffic situation to ensure scene safety?

(A) Continue to let the traffic flow as it is so that the road remains open.
(B) Divert the traffic around the scene, allowing cars to pass.
(C) Completely block traffic flow until the operations are complete.
(D) Detour the traffic from the main roadway at the previous exit.

693. Which of the following statements is incorrect concerning confined space rescue?

(A) Confined space rescuers may encounter hazardous atmospheres.

(B) Confined space rescuers may encounter a potential for engulfment.

(C) Exposed electrical wiring may be a hidden danger to the rescuer.

(D) Paramedics may enter a confined space without safety equipment as long as they are accompanied by trained rescuers.

694. All of the following are conditions in which the sacrifice of initial definitive patient care to provide extrication would be acceptable in order to ensure final positive patient outcome EXCEPT

(A) a patient trapped in a car which was pinned up against a tree in a flash flood with a rapidly rising water level

(B) a patient pinned in a car under a leaking gasoline tanker

(C) a patient who has fallen from a cliff side and is at the bottom of a steep slope

(D) a chemical worker lying unconscious in a chemical holding tank

695. You are called to the scene of a 32-year-old male who was last seen crawling into a dense area of brush. On your arrival, his friends explain that he wanted to "check out" this thick area for nesting animals. It has been about an hour since he was last seen. What should you request from communications to assist you in this search?

(A) helicopter support with high-intensity lighting

(B) specially trained dogs and experienced search managers

(C) a high-angle rescue team

(D) four-wheel drive vehicles

696. You respond to the scene of a car that hit a pole. Upon your arrival, you notice that the power lines are down on the top of the vehicle and the occupants are still inside. When would you consider it safe to operate within the area of the downed power line?

(A) when the power line stops sparking

(B) when the fire department arrives and moves the power line off the vehicle with a hook

(C) when the patient's condition warrants a rapid extrication

(D) when the local power company arrives on scene and advises that power has been cut to that line

697. Which of the following vehicles should be considered unstable to operate in until properly stabilized?

(A) an overturned vehicle
(B) a vehicle that has hit a wall
(C) a vehicle that has struck a bridge support
(D) All vehicles are considered unstable until properly supported.

698. You are on the scene of a one-car collision, and the vehicle is leaking gasoline. You also notice a build-up of gasoline fumes in the area. All of the following should be done to decrease the possibility of an explosion and subsequent fire EXCEPT

(A) cutting the battery cable
(B) turning off the ignition
(C) securing the area of all bystanders
(D) minimizing the use of tools that may cause sparks

699. Your patient is trapped inside a vehicle that was hit in the driver's door. To gain access and remove your patient from the vehicle, which of the following should be done first?

(A) Have the extrication team come in and open the door with a power tool.
(B) Break the glass and enter the vehicle through the window, and then alert the extrication team.
(C) Try the undamaged door on the other side to see if will offer access.
(D) Remove the roof of the vehicle.

700. Your patient has fallen off a bridge and is trapped on a rock in rapidly moving water. Your initial rescue attempt should be to

(A) Attempt to reach the patient only after you are secured to a rope.
(B) Try to climb down to the patient from the bridge.
(C) Alert a swift-water rescue team and stand by until they arrive.
(D) Don a life vest and attempt to swim to the patient.

701. All of the following situations would require immediate removal prior to a full assessment and proper stabilization EXCEPT

(A) a patient in a vehicle that was involved in a head-on collision
(B) a patient who is in a tank and overcome by toxic gases
(C) a patient who is trapped in a collapsed trench
(D) a patient who is inside a burning vehicle but complaining of numbness in his or her extremities

702. The greatest hazard of a deployed supplemental restraint system (SRS), or airbag, is

(A) The inflated SRS will hinder airway management interventions.
(B) The deployed SRS has a residue on it that may cause burns.
(C) The deployed SRS will reduce the area in which the rescuer has to operate.
(D) The deployed SRS will produce no hazard to the rescuer.

703. If the rescuer is exposed to the SRS lubricant, what is the appropriate intervention to eliminate the possibility of burns?

(A) The rescuer should thoroughly wash all exposed areas as soon as possible.

(B) The rescuer should seek treatment in the emergency department for possible treatment of irritation.

(C) Rescuers who have come in contact with SRS should contact poison control for further instructions.

(D) As this is a toxic chemical, all rescuers should be completely decontaminated after coming in contact with an SRS.

704. Which of the following should NOT be done in a situation in which a vehicle was in a collision and the SRS has not deployed?

(A) Disconnect the battery cable.

(B) Avoid placing body in the direct path of a possibly deploying SRS.

(C) Avoid placing any heat in the area of the steering wheel hub.

(D) Drill into the SRS module to release the charge.

705. All of the following are aspects of prolonged patient care by the Paramedic during extended rescue efforts EXCEPT

(A) on-scene amputation of limbs to initiate rescue on critical patients

(B) cleansing and wound care

(C) pain management

(D) removal of impaled objects

706. You arrive at the scene of a car that has been driven over the side of a ravine. You call for additional resources, which include a specially trained team of rescuers who can gain access to the patient. This type of rescue is known as

(A) rappelling rescue

(B) vertical rescue

(C) team rescue

(D) technical rescue

707. The Paramedic's main objective when encountering an entrapped patient is disentanglement and treatment. Which of the following best describes disentanglement?

(A) mitigation of all scene hazards to ensure rapid extrication

(B) removal of the patient from the entrapping section of the vehicle

(C) removal of the entrapping section of the vehicle from the patient

(D) the effort of the Paramedic to avoid becoming trapped in the vehicle with the patient

708. You and your partner are called to the scene of a police officer who has been shot. On your arrival, you are told that the gunman has barricaded himself in his house and a police officer has been shot. The officer is located on the front lawn in direct view of the gunman. The commander at the scene informs you that he will provide you with a "cover" team to assist you in the extrication of the wounded police officer from the lawn. You should

(A) Prepare your equipment for a rapid patient removal.

(B) Advise the commander that you are not trained in tactical rescue and await his decision.

(C) Attempt to talk with the gunman to "make a deal" in order to remove the policeman.

(D) Protect yourself and your partner by refusing this assignment, since it could lead to additional casualties.

709. One of the primary means of gaining information for rapidly locating patients trapped in a building collapse is

(A) interviewing witnesses and building employees for building occupancy areas

(B) performing a rapid, blind search of the building

(C) sending in large independent teams to sweep all areas

(D) alerting the proper agencies for specialized equipment to locate trapped building occupants

710. A major concern for the Paramedic while treating a patient who has been removed after being trapped by heavy debris in a building collapse is

(A) open fractures

(B) rapid cardiovascular collapse

(C) cavitation injuries

(D) impaled objects

RESCUE AWARENESS

A N S W E R S

691. The answer is B. (Mosby/ACEP, *General Principles of Rescue*.) (B) Securing hazardous materials leaks is not the primary role of the Paramedic. Paramedics are a patient care resource, and their primary role includes the following: (A) evaluation of scene safety, searching for the location of all patients, patient count; and resources; (C) gaining access to and initial care of the patient; (D) extrication and continued care; and, finally, transportation of the patient. Personnel who are untrained in hazardous materials mitigation should never attempt to secure a hazardous materials scene.

692. The answer is C. (Mosby/ACEP, *General Principles of Rescue*.) (C) The complete blocking of a roadway is always the safest choice in providing scene safety. Blocking the roadway will result in the complete stoppage of traffic and eliminate any chance of a secondary accident caused by passing vehicles. You should never operate while you (A) continue to let traffic flow normally, since this poses a major hazard to the rescuers at the scene. (B) Diversion of traffic around the scene still poses a risk to rescuers, although it is an option. (D) Rescuers may detour traffic at the previous exit; however, on a major highway, the exits may be separated by many miles of road, which would still leave vehicles heading in your direction at high speeds.

693. The answer is D. (Brady, *Rescue Operations*.) (D) Untrained and unequipped Paramedics should never enter a confined space without training or equipment. The fact that they are with trained team members does nothing for their personal safety. Rescuers may encounter (A) hazardous atmospheres, specifically, low oxygen levels and toxins. Paramedics also run the risk of (B) potential for engulfment by falling debris, grain, and other materials at the scene. (C) Exposed electrical wiring may also be an inherent danger to the untrained rescuer. Untrained Paramedics should remain outside the danger area until the rescue team extricates the patient to the treatment area.

694. The answer is C. (Brady, *Rescue Operations.*) (C) The patient who is at the bottom of a steep slope will not pose any major risk to rescuers should they delay extrication for initial care. Patients who are (A) trapped in fast moving water are in a situation that cannot be stabilized by rescue workers, as are patients who are (B) pinned under leaking containers of flammable liquids or (D) exposed to chemical substances. These patients will all benefit from their removal from the danger prior to the initiation of definitive care.

695. The answer is B. (Brady, *The Rescue Operation.*) (B) In thick brush, even the most well-trained rescuer could be easily disoriented. The use of search dogs may be required to track the movements of your patient. Although (A) helicopters with high-intensity lighting are usually a great asset, if the patient is lost in thick brush, it is possible that the helicopter will have no visibility of the ground. (C) A high-angle rescue team is not required, since you are in brush and not dealing with angles, hills, and slopes. (D) Four-wheel drive vehicles will not work in thick brush. This is a slow-moving, coordinated search using dogs and/or sensitive equipment for location of the patient.

696. The answer is D. (Caroline, *Rescue and Extrication.*) (D) The Paramedic should never attempt to operate in the presence of power lines. Paramedics should request the local power company to respond to the scene and have the power shut down. (A) A power line that is not sparking is not an indicator of its status. (B) Although many fire departments will remove a power line from a vehicle, this is in no way a guarantee that the area is safe; the line could contact water or even send its charge through wet grass, creating a dangerous condition for rescue personnel. (C) The patient's condition will have no bearing on the approach to a charged area. The standard rule is safety of the rescuer first, and it should not be broken at any time.

697. The answer is D. (Caroline, *Rescue and Extrication.*) (D) The Paramedic should consider even the most harmless-looking vehicle unstable until it is properly supported. While (A) overturned vehicles, (B) vehicles crashed into walls, and (C) vehicles that have struck a bridge support all have their own inherent dangers, the vehicle that is on all four tires and even terrain should be checked and stabilized prior to entry.

698. The answer is A. (Caroline, *Rescue and Extrication.*) (A) The battery cable should never be cut in this situation. Cables tend to create sparks when cut, and the possibility of grounding out the vehicle always exists. The Paramedic should ensure that (B) the ignition is in the off position, (C) the area is secured from all bystanders who could compound the problem by creating unnecessary hazards (e.g., smoking, etc.), and (D) the minimal use of tools that may cause a spark should be considered.

699. The answer is C. (Caroline, *Rescue and Extrication.*) (C) Sometimes the simplest solution is the one that is the most logical. If the passenger door will open, you will have eliminated inherent dangers of power tools as well as saved valuable time in the care of your patient. (A) Power tools should be used when other means of access are unsuccessful. (B) Breaking the glass is used to enter the vehicle when long extrication may be forthcoming, but patients are not removed through windows of the vehicle. (D) It is common to have the roof removed during an extrication; however, if the passenger door opens, use the easiest solution.

700. **The answer is C.** (Brady, *Rescue Operations.*) (C) The Paramedic should alert a swift-water rescue team immediately if he or she is not trained to accomplish this type of rescue. Swift-water rescue requires extensive experience and should not be attempted by one who has no training. (A), (B), and (D) are all incorrect, since they all compromise rescuer safety.

701. **The answer is A.** (Brady, *Rescue Operations.*) (A) Although the patient who has been in a head-on collision could be quite critical, if there are no hazards involved, this patient would warrant a full assessment as well as proper stabilization. The patient who is (B) overcome by toxic gases in a tank will benefit from immediate extrication from the area. Patients who are (C) trapped in a collapsed trench will also benefit from immediate extrication for fear of further collapse. (D) Patients, although possibly suffering from spinal injury, are in extreme danger from burn injury when trapped inside a burning vehicle. These patients will benefit from basic immobilization and rapid extrication from harm's way.

702. **The answer is B.** (Mosby, *Rescue Management.*) (B) The deployed SRS contains either cornstarch or talcum powder mixed with sodium hydroxide, which will cause nonhazardous irritation to unprotected skin. Rescuers should wear glove and eye protection while operating near deployed SRS. (A) and (C) are incorrect, since the SRS does not remain inflated. (D) is incorrect, since the SRS does produce some hazard to the rescuer, as described in answer (B).

703. **The answer is A.** (Mosby, *Rescue Management.*) Rescuers who have exposed skin come in contact with SRS lubricant (A) should wash thoroughly after contact as soon as possible to remove all of the SRS lubricant. Severe burns are usually never involved with SRS deployment, so (B) treatment at an emergency department is not indicated. (C) and (D) are incorrect, since this lubricant is not an extremely toxic exposure and does not require poison control or decontamination interventions.

704. **The answer is D.** (Mosby, *Rescue Management.*) (D) The rescuer should never drill into an SRS module; this action could deploy the SRS system and injure the rescuer as well as the patient. (A), (B), and (C) are all proper operating procedures for an undeployed SRS.

705. **The answer is A.** (Brady, *The Rescue Operation.*) (A) Although amputation in the field to ensure the survival of the patient is a possibility, it is not within the Paramedic's scope of practice and should be accomplished by an on-scene physician. There are many additions to management of the critical patient who is in need of disentanglement. These include answers (B), (C), and (D).

706. The answer is B. (Brady, *The Rescue Operation*.) (B) Anytime a rescue team must contend with the forces of gravity, the operation is known as a vertical rescue. These specially trained teams require special equipment and constant training to effect a successful rescue. The untrained and unequipped Paramedic should not attempt these types of rescues. (A), (C), and (D) are all aspects of this type of rescue. Rappelling is used to gain access; it is a team effort, and it is certainly a technical rescue, but it is also part of the picture of a vertical rescue and not its definition.

707. The answer is C. (Caroline, *Rescue and Extrication*.) (C) Removal of the entrapping section of the vehicle is the primary objective of disentanglement. The Paramedic should not attempt to (B) remove the patient from the entrapping section prior to the section's being cleared. These actions could cause additional injuries to the patient. (A) is incorrect, although all scene hazards should be cleared prior to beginning the extrication and disentanglement effort. (D) does not describe disentanglement, although it does fall into the scene-safety category.

708. The answer is D. (Mosby/ACEP, *General Principles of Rescue*.) (D) At no time should an untrained rescuer move into the line of fire. Rescuer safety is of the highest priority and remains so in this situation. Most police departments have (B) tactical Paramedics who are trained in these situations and will remove the patient for you; police departments also have their own negotiators who will (C) talk to the gunman to remedy the situation. At no time should the rescuer (A) prepare to enter this area.

709. The answer is A. (Mosby/ACEP, *General Principles of Rescue*.) (A) Witness interviews are essential in the location of large building use areas. These interviews can assist the rescuer in understanding exactly where the highest occupancy areas of the building are. (B) A rapid, blind search of the building with a plan could slow down rescue efforts. (C) Large independent teams will also hinder the effort with their lack of communications. Small teams should be sent in and should be in constant communication with each other. (D) Specialized equipment will be needed in these situations, but rescue efforts should not be delayed awaiting their arrival.

710. The answer is B. (Mosby/ACEP, *General Principles of Rescue*.) (B) Cardiovascular collapse and subsequent cardiac arrest are the primary concerns for a patient with crush syndrome after a building collapse. Acidosis and hyperkalemia should be treated immediately to prevent this occurrence. Although (A) open fractures, (C) cavitation injuries, and (D) impaled objects all require priority management, treatment and maintenance of cardiovascular function are of the highest priority.

HAZARDOUS MATERIALS

Directions: Each item below contains four suggested responses. Select the **one best** response to each item.

711. All of the following are responsibilities of the hazardous materials first responder EXCEPT

    (A) knowledge of hazardous materials and the risks associated with them in case of an accident

    (B) the ability to recognize the need for specialty resources

    (C) an understanding of the potential outcomes of a hazardous materials emergency

    (D) entry to the hot zone and mitigation of the incident

712. You respond to an overturned truck on a busy freeway. On your arrival, you notice that the truck has a placard that has white and red stripes. This truck is most likely carrying

    (A) flammable liquids

    (B) flammable solids

    (C) explosives

    (D) oxidizers

713. The guidebook that the EMS responder would most likely use to identify a hazardous material by its UN number as well as obtain safety information is

    (A) DOT emergency response guidebook

    (B) a Paramedic hazardous materials textbook

    (C) DOT truck placard chart

    (D) the shipper's manifest

714. All EMS operations at a hazardous materials incident should take place in the

    (A) hot zone

    (B) warm zone

    (C) cold zone

    (D) wherever the largest number of patients are

715. While on the scene of a hazardous materials incident, in order to get additional information regarding a specific chemical product (agent), the responder may call

(A) FEMA
(B) the Centers for Disease Control
(C) CHEMTREC
(D) poison control

716. The type of personal protective equipment that provides the highest level of protection at a hazardous materials incident is known as

(A) level A
(B) level B
(C) level C
(D) level D

717. The initial approach to a chemically contaminated patient should include

(A) a complete history and physical examination
(B) pharmacological intervention
(C) cardiac monitoring
(D) assessment of the ABCs, cervical spine management, and decontamination

718. The OSHA requirement that all members of a hazardous materials entry team receive a complete assessment prior to and after "suiting up" is known as

(A) team assessment
(B) medical surveillance
(C) provider guidelines
(D) DOT protection clause

HAZARDOUS MATERIALS

ANSWERS

711. **The answer is D.** (Mosby, *Hazardous Materials.*) (D) Hazardous materials first responders are not trained in the mitigation of a hazardous materials incident. Hazardous materials technicians and specialists accomplish mitigation. The first responder is responsible for (A) knowledge of the risks associated with hazardous materials, (B) the ability to recognize the need for special resources, and (C) an understanding of potential outcomes. Hazardous materials first responders are responsible to protect nearby life, property, and environmental issues. They do not attempt to control the release of the agent.

712. **The answer is B.** (Mosby/ACEP, *Hazardous Materials and Radiation Incidents.*) (B) The DOT placard system identifies flammable solids with a white and red striped placard. The EMS responder should be aware that shippers are only required to place a placard on a vehicle if it is carrying more than 1001 pounds of an agent. Responders should take great caution in approaching any shipping container that has no placard. (A), (C), and (D) are incorrect.

713. **The answer is A.** (Mosby/ACEP, *Hazardous Materials and Radiation Incidents.*) (A) The DOT emergency response guidebook will allow the first responding vehicle to identify the type of hazardous material involved in the incident, as well as obtain information on safety distances and evacuation. It will also give basic emergency care information to the provider to assist in patient care. (B) Although a Paramedic textbook may have good information on hazardous materials, it will usually not have specific information on all materials. (C) The DOT placard chart explains the types of agents but does not break it down into specifics. (D) The shipper's manifest is an excellent resource for the cargo information, but it may not be readily available during an emergency. If the driver is injured or unconscious, or there is a leak of product, the provider will not have access to the manifest.

714. **The answer is C.** (Mosby, *Hazardous Materials*.) (C) All EMS operations are to be provided in the cold zone to patients after they are decontaminated. Individuals properly trained in personal protective equipment should do decontamination. Decontamination is usually done in the warm zone with a corridor into the cold zone. EMS providers should remain in the cold zone regardless of the situation at the scene unless they are properly trained and outfitted in personal protective equipment. (A) Hot zone is the actual incident. (B) Warm zone requires personal protective equipment and is usually set up as a decontamination area. (D) The patient locations have no effect on the location of the cold zone.

715. **The answer is C.** (Mosby, *Hazardous Materials*.) (C) CHEMTREC is a 24-hour hotline designed to provide trained experts to assist in hazardous materials incident mitigation. A call to 1-800-CHEMTREC will allow responders to obtain comprehensive information regarding specific chemicals and their effects on the body. CHEMTREC will also provide fire officials with information on product mitigation and decontamination. (A), (B), and (D) are all incorrect.

716. **The answer is A.** (Mosby/ACEP, *Hazardous Materials and Radiation Incidents*.) (A) Level A protection provides a fully encapsulating chemical resistant suit with self-contained breathing apparatus. (B) Level B provides the same respiratory protection but not the same mucous membrane protection. (C) Level C provides an air-purifying respirator and chemical-resistant clothing. (D) Level D provides no respiratory protection and minimal mucous membrane protection.

717. **The answer is D.** (Mosby/ACEP, *Hazardous Materials and Radiation Incidents*.) (D) The treatment of a chemically contaminated patient should be minimized to airway, breathing, and circulation, and cervical spine maintenance prior to decontamination. It is important to stress that the Paramedic should not be in contact with contaminated patients unless he or she is trained in the use of personal protective equipment. After the patient is decontaminated, the Paramedic should (A) take a complete history and perform a physical examination, (B) begin pharmacological intervention, and (C) monitor the ECG for any irregularities.

718. **The answer is B.** (Mosby/ACEP, *Hazardous Materials and Radiation Incidents*.) (B) Medical surveillance is conducted on all members of an entry team prior to suiting up in personal protective equipment. This physical includes assessment of pulse, temperature, respiration, blood pressure, cardiac rhythm, weight, cognitive and motor skills, and hydration. This assessment is done after exit to determine whether the provider is or is not capable of reentry to the scene. (A), (C), and (D) are all incorrect.

BIBLIOGRAPHY

Bledsoe BE, Porter RS, Shade BR: *Paramedic Emergency Care.* Upper Saddle River, NJ, Brady, Prentice-Hall, 1997.

Caroline NR: *Emergency Care in the Streets.* Boston, Little Brown, 1995.

Cason D, Pons PT: *Paramedic Field Care.* St. Louis, Mosby-Lifeline and the American College of Emergency Physicians, 1997.

Sanders MJ: *Mosby's Paramedic Textbook.* St. Louis, Mosby-Lifeline, 1994.

NOTES

NOTES

NOTES

NOTES

NOTES

NOTES

NOTES

NOTES

NOTES

NOTES

ISBN 0-07-134156-0